FULL
OF
LIFE

LUC DE SCHEPPER
M.D., Ph.D., Lic. Ac.

TALE WEAVER
PUBLISHING

LOS ANGELES

1st Printing

Library of Congress Catalog Card Number: 91-075086

ISBN 0-942139-12-7

Printed in the United States of America

The information in this book is not intended as medical advice. Its intention is solely informational and educational. It is assumed that the reader will consult a medical or health professional should the need for one be warranted.

Tale Weaver Publishing, Los Angeles, CA 90069

Dedicated to my wife
Yolanda and mom Betty.

ACKNOWLEDGMENTS

A work like this is the result of love and teamwork between doctor and patient. Therefore, all my patients have contributed to this book. The drawings are the result of the talents of Shay Marlowe and my beloved Yolanda. I want to thank the president and vice president of Tale Weaver, Dick Weaver and the late Ron Baron, for believing in this project and for giving their invaluable professional advice. Working with my editor, Gretchen Henkel, was not only a pleasure but also a learning experience. Lucy Mack Bryant with her wonderful insight was my best critic in the most positive way. And David Horowitz (Author of *The Kennedy's*) was a wonderful support and friend to help me out in any way he could. Without the help of my mother-in-law, Betty, who helped me type the whole manuscript, I could not have brought out this book on time.

Anyone afflicted by these diseases should consult a nutritional, holistically oriented doctor. I want to thank my patients for confiding in me, for working with me and showing their confidence and hope. Without them, this book would not be possible. I feel fortunate to have my patients as my friends, for having taught so much about suffering, compassion and love. Hopefully, this book will give hope to millions of sufferers and a return to a healthy, fulfilling life.

Luc De Schepper M.D., Ph.D., Lic. Ac.
2901 Wilshire Blvd, Ste 435
Santa Monica, CA 90403
Tel: (213) 828-4480

TABLE OF CONTENTS

SECTION THREE: TREATMENTS AND BEYOND: REGAINING HEALTH AND ACHIEVING PEAK IMMUNITY

SECTION ONE

A NEW UNDERSTANDING OF HEALTH AND IMMUNITY

INTRODUCTION

Wouldn't it be great to wake up each morning with energy to spare? Wouldn't you like to feel full of life every day? Of course, we all would. But this isn't just some idle wish. Achieving peak immunity is within your power. Read this book, follow its guidelines, and you'll have more energy than you believed possible.

Some of you already know that things aren't right with your health. Others may suspect that something is wrong, but may be hesitant to say just what they are experiencing. And then there are still others who are certain that they've got nothing to worry about.

What is happening to our health? If you look at national statistics, we are in a health crisis of epidemic proportions. For the last decade, we have watched the unfolding of the AIDS epidemic; in the same period, more and more seemingly young and vigorous adults have been suffering from chronic fatigue, and people on the whole seem more prone to develop viral and other chronic illnesses. Is there something we can do about it? The answer in this book is a resounding YES!

Whether you're perfectly healthy right now, or ill with CFIDS (Chronic Fatigue Immune Dysfunction Syndrome), you can use the information here to make your life better by achieving peak immunity.

This book takes a new look at the concepts of health and illness. When you can see your symptoms in the context of a bigger picture, as signs of how your immune system is working, then you can begin to make the kinds of changes that will be long-lasting. If you are suffering from CFIDS or your immune system is not functioning at a peak level, be assured that you can get better. Ultimately, we all need to think in terms of preventing illness rather than waiting until it happens to cure it. For some practitioners, this has always been the goal. With the help of this book, it can become your goal too. With the information and therapy plans outlined here, you can become an effective partner in your own health care.

In the 90s, the physician will become a lifestyle expert and wellness adviser. Patients will be treated as whole beings, not just as collections of symptoms. Non-invasive diagnostic procedures, such as MRI (magnetic resonance imaging) and ultrasound, are tools that have already revolutionized medicine. They will continue to arm physicians with information, allowing them to prescribe preventive measures as well as treatments for latent, undiagnosed conditions. Psychoimmunology, a new medical field which considers the role of the emotions in physical well-being, will become vitally important.

As you will see in the chapters that follow, it will take more than some new "magic bullets" to repair the damage done to the complex systems in your body that protect you from disease. None of the immuno-suppressed conditions discussed here can be corrected without taking lifestyle, dietary and environmental factors into account.

Here is a thumbnail sketch of what has happened, a summary of the changes in the conditions of our lives that have produced this crisis of health:

* In the first place, we have changed what we eat. Take a quick look at the American diet. It is low in fiber, low in high-quality, low-fat protein and high in sugars, simple carbohydrates and fat. If food and drinks do not taste sweet, we add chemicals like saccharin and Nutrasweet ™. The results of the modern diet are devastating: atherosclerotic heart disease and stroke, hypertension, colon cancer, obesity, dental cavities and many other diseases are rampant.

* Technology has also proved to be a two-edged sword. The introduction of many miracle drugs has aided us in the battle against disease. But others have resulted in addictions, immuno-suppressed conditions and a whole array of new diseases.

* Stress and pressure dominate our lifestyles. Just when we thought that the high technology we created would bring us more free time, more joy and relaxation, the contrary is the case. We

seem to feel obliged to work longer hours. Career goals dominate the household picture and spouses forget how to communicate with each other. Modern living has become high-stress living. Emotional traumas and daily stress are THE triggering factors in the suppression of the immune system.

The key to fighting off disease is a healthy immune system. How do you know if yours is functioning well? You can find out by taking the self-scoring questionnaire in Chapter One. You might be suffering from a pre-condition that can lead to the debilitating Chronic Fatigue Immune Dysfunction Syndrome (1) and/or other immune suppressing illnesses.

In the following pages, there is an outline of how the immune system works, and how you can protect it and keep it strong, so that it, in turn, can take good care of you and keep you healthy throughout a lifetime. This book will help you to determine, with the help of your doctor, what's wrong with you; it will provide you with natural treatments to combat lethargy and boost your immune system. The book will also teach you how to handle the stress of any chronic disease, and CFIDS in particular. May the knowledge of this book put you on the road to peak immunity!

Footnote:
1. The most recent name for this condition is Chronic Fatigue and Immune Dysfunction Syndrome (CFIDS) in the United States or Myalgic Encephalitis (M.E.) in the U.K. and Australia.

CHAPTER ONE

ARE YOU AT RISK
FOR DECREASED IMMUNITY OR HEALTH?

Are you as healthy as you want to be? Are you visiting your doctor more often, but still not feeling any better? Do you want to have more energy?

You are not alone. Despite incredible advances by medical science, Americans seem to be suffering from a multitude of new diseases and conditions.

Thanks to antibiotics and powerful vaccines such as the polio vaccine, we no longer lose victims to such diseases as scarlet fever or poliomyelitis. But there are new viruses and syndromes plaguing our population. Why are AIDS (Acquired Immune Deficiency Syndrome) and CFIDS (Chronic Fatigue Immune Dysfunction syndrome) so prevalent now? What has happened to our general state of health that these debilitating conditions are taking hold?

This book explores the answers to these and other questions, and gives you real therapies and guidelines for changing the course of your own health.

But before you read any further, you need to know the status of your immune system. Take the following self-scoring questionnaire. It contains lots of questions about your heredity, environmental influences, and symptoms that, combined in frequent enough proportions, can indicate that you could be at risk or are already suffering from an immuno-suppressed condition.

A word of caution here. A self-scoring questionnaire, such as the one designed here, is not intended to be a scientific diagnostic tool. Its goal is merely to bring your attention to a possible problem and encourage you to seek help from a doctor.

SELF-SCORING QUESTIONNAIRE

This self-scoring test consists of two parts. The first part is designed to illuminate the triggering factors that can lead to a weakened immune system. The second part pinpoints symptoms and signs of a compromised immune system.

Completing this questionnaire will give you a good indication of the state of your immune system. Read the questions carefully and answer them as honestly as possible. It's in your own best interest to get an accurate reading. Part One relies on yes or no answers, with scoring instructions for each section. Part Two uses a relative rating system. Once you have completed all the questions, obtain the scoring from the end of the questionnaire and add up your total score. Then see the end of this section for your corresponding wellness category.

A. TRIGGERING FACTORS

Your family history and your personality type can often predispose you for immune system problems. The following questions are designed to pinpoint the presence of these factors in your life.

Your Heredity

Has one of your parents or any of your siblings suffered from one of the following diseases?

1. Manic-depressive disorder   Yes _____ No _____

2. Diabetes   Yes _____ No _____

3. Rheumatoid Arthritis (R.A.)   Yes _____ No _____

4. Low thyroid function   Yes _____ No _____

5. Cancer in any form   Yes _____ No _____

6. Hypoglycemia   Yes _____ No _____

7. Allergies   Yes _____ No _____

8. Lupus Erythematosus (S.L.E.)   Yes _____ No _____

9. Multiple Sclerosis (M.S.)   Yes _____ No _____

Your Personality

10. Are you highly competitive?   Yes _____ No _____

11. Are you impatient and driven?   Yes _____ No _____

12. Is your hostility easily aroused?   Yes _____ No _____

13. Are you obsessive about exercise?   Yes _____ No _____

14. Are you nervous and easily frustrated?   Yes _____ No _____

15. Do you judge your accomplishments in concrete terms, i.e., material possessions, how much money you make, etc.?   Yes _____ No _____

16. Do you have difficulty taking time for genuine relaxation?
Yes _____ No _____

17. Are you aggressive?   Yes _____ No _____

18. Are you extroverted?   Yes _____ No _____

19. Do you dominate conversations?   Yes _____ No _____

20. Are you insecure about yourself?   Yes _____ No _____

21. Do you hate to be disliked?   Yes _____ No _____

22. Are you hard-working?   Yes _____ No _____

23. Are you overly analytical?   Yes _____ No _____

24. Are you obsessed with the past?   Yes _____ No _____

Stressful Life Events

Any change, positive or negative, in your life situation can be stressful. According to research pioneered by social scientists

Holmes and Rahe, too many stressful events in the same time period can leave you vulnerable to illness. Again, answer the questions with a "yes" or "no."

Have you recently (within the last year) experienced:

25. Death of your spouse?   Yes _____ No _____

26. Divorce?   Yes _____ No _____

27. Death of a close family member?   Yes _____ No _____

28. Marital separation?   Yes _____ No _____

29. Jail term?   Yes _____ No _____

30. Personal injury? Yes _____ No _____

31. A new marriage?   Yes _____ No _____

32. Dismissal from your job?   Yes _____ No _____

33. Retirement?   Yes _____ No _____

34. Pregnancy?   Yes _____ No _____

35. Difficulties with sex?   Yes _____ No _____

36. Mortgage or loan over $100,000?   Yes _____ No _____

37. Trouble with in-laws?   Yes _____ No _____

38. Trouble with your boss?   Yes _____ No _____

39. Change in residence, working hours, habits or other routine activities?   Yes _____ No _____

40. Were you in the past the victim of child-abuse?   Yes ___ No ___

41. Were one or both of your parents alcoholics?   Yes _____ No _____

Nutritional Factors

As with the section above, answer "yes" or "no" to each question, then see the end of the questionnaire for scoring.

42. Are you addicted to sugar, Nutrasweet ™, or chocolate? Yes _____ No _____

43. Do you drink diet soft drinks regularly?   Yes _____ No _____

44. Do you binge on particular foods?   Yes _____ No _____

45. Do you have an increased intake of raw food (eating at salad bars or sushi restaurants)?   Yes _____ No _____

46. Do you have cravings for bread?   Yes _____ No _____

47. Do you regularly omit eating breakfast?   Yes _____ No _____

48. Do you eat products containing white flour?   Yes _____ No _____

49. Do you have irregular eating habits?   Yes _____ No _____

50. Do you eat a lot of fried foods?   Yes _____ No _____

51. Do you rarely eat grains such as brown rice, wild rice, buckwheat, quinoa, amaranth or millet?   Yes _____ No _____

52. Does your diet consist mainly of carbohydrates, especially simple ones (potatoes, bread, pasta, etc.)?   Yes _____ No _____

53. Do you consume alcoholic beverages regularly? Yes _____ No _____

54. Are you addicted to coffee?   Yes _____ No _____

55. Are you overweight?   Yes _____ No _____

56. Do you have a lot of food allergies?   Yes _____ No _____

57. Do you eat pork regularly?   Yes _____ No _____

58. Do you rarely eat fresh fruits?   Yes _____ No _____

Exterior Factors

Answer the questions in this section with a "yes" or "no," then turn to the end of the questionnaire for point scoring.

Have you ever been subjected to:

59. Operations?   Yes _____ No _____

60. Intake of cytostatica (anti-cancer medication, or radiation treatments?   Yes _____ No _____

Have you ever taken:

61. Tetracycline for treatment of acne (for at least two months or longer)?   Yes _____ No _____

62. Cortisone, either orally or by injection?   Yes _____ No _____

63. Antibiotics, especially broad-spectrum (Keflex, Bactrim, Ampicillin)?   Yes _____ No _____

64. Have you used or are you using marijuana, cocaine or heroin?   Yes _____ No _____

65. Do you smoke cigarettes?   Yes _____ No _____

66. Have you had recurrent viral or bacterial infections - more than six in a year?   Yes _____ No _____

67. Have you ever taken birth control pills, for at least a year or longer?   Yes _____ No _____

Do you feel worse:

68. When you are exposed to ragweed/pollen?   Yes _____ No _____

69. When you rake leaves?   Yes _____ No _____

70. When you are in a damp basement?   Yes _____ No _____

71. Do you increasingly feel more uncomfortable with your environment (reacting to smoke, fumes, perfumes, pesticides, and a resulting inability to visit public places)?   Yes _____ No _____

Are you subjected to any of the following chemical stressors in your home?

72. Aluminum pots and pans?   Yes _____ No _____

73. Ammonia?   Yes _____ No _____

74. Fluoridated water?   Yes _____ No _____

75. Dyes?   Yes _____ No _____

76. Gas stoves or heaters?   Yes _____ No _____

77. Hair sprays?   Yes _____ No _____

78. Kerosene?   Yes _____ No _____

79. Lacquer?   Yes _____ No _____

80. Teflon pots and pans?   Yes _____ No _____

81. Turpentine?   Yes _____ No _____

82. Paint fumes?   Yes _____ No _____

83. Newspaper print?   Yes _____ No _____

84. Nail polish?   Yes _____ No _____

85. Pesticides?   Yes _____ No _____

86. Tobacco smoke?   Yes _____ No _____

87. Formaldehyde?   Yes _____ No _____

88. Are you living or have you ever lived in a damp climate for at least one year (foggy beach, damp states such as New York, Florida, Oregon or Washington, D.C.)?   Yes _____ No _____

89. Have you ever experienced adverse reactions to any medications or drugs?   Yes _____ No _____

Immediately after exposure, do any of the following items make you feel physically ill or have an emotional effect on you? (I.e., do you experience depression or mood swings immediately after exposure?)

90. Mold, mildew?   Yes _____ No _____

91. Dust?   Yes _____ No _____

92. Cats, dogs?   Yes _____ No _____

93. Gas?   Yes _____ No _____

94. Cigarettes?   Yes _____ No _____

95. Bleaches?   Yes _____ No _____

96. Paint?   Yes _____ No _____

97. Dyes?   Yes _____ No _____

98. Gasoline?   Yes _____ No _____

99. Insecticides?   Yes _____ No _____

Do you work in a building with:

100. Inadequate lighting?   Yes _____ No _____

101. Inadequate windows in your working area?   Yes _____ No _____

102. Recycled air?   Yes _____ No _____

103. Parking underneath the building?   Yes _____ No _____

104. Ceilings containing asbestos?   Yes _____ No _____

105. Regular lighting (absence of full spectrum lights)?
Yes _____ No _____

106. Smoking permitted? Yes _____ No _____

107. Many copying machines, X-ray equipment or computers
present?   Yes _____ No _____

B. SYMPTOMS

Grade the following symptoms according to severity, using these
abbreviations:

Never:	N
Occasional:	O
Moderate:	M
Severe:	S

After grading the symptoms, turn to the end of this questionnaire
for point scoring.

Brain Symptoms

108. Difficulty concentrating, inability to stay with the thread of a
conversation _____

109. Decreased short-term memory (memory for recent events,
forgetful about friends' names, feeling of an early stage of Alzheimer's
disease) _____

110. Drowsiness throughout the day. _____

111. Dyslexia and difficulty with easy calculations (balancing one's
checkbook, for instance). _____

112. Headaches _____

113. Severe mood swings _____

114. Suicidal thoughts _____

115. Anger and irritability ____

116. Frustration ____

Hormonal Symptoms

117. Premenstrual syndrome (PMS) ____

118. Flareup of yeast infections the week before the menstrual cycle or immediately after intercourse ____

119. Loss of sexual desire ____

120. Impotence ____

121. Endometriosis ____

122. Menstrual irregularities ____

123. Early menopause ____

Digestive Symptoms

124. Gas ____

125. Abdominal distention ____

126. Diarrhea ____

127. Constipation ____

128. Hemorrhoids ____

129. Abdominal pain ____

130. Mucus in the stool ____

131. Greenish stools ____

132. Anal itching ____

133. Heartburn ____

134. Bad breath _____

135. Constant hungry feeling _____

136. Weight loss or gain without a change of diet _____

137. Presence of a thick, yellow fur in the middle of the tongue, especially in the morning _____

138. Food allergies _____

Other Symptoms

139. Recurrent colds - five or more in one year _____

140. Recurrent urinary tract infections, especially after sexual intercourse _____

141. Recurrent sore throats and swollen glands _____

142. Persistent fatigue _____

143. Sneezing spells _____

144. Hay fever _____

145. Postnasal drip _____

146. Cold limbs _____

147. Joint and muscle pain _____

148. Itching _____

149. Hives _____

150. Runny nose _____

151. Earaches _____

152. Hoarseness _____

153. Intermittent fevers ____

154. Dizziness and unsteadiness, especially when changing body positions ____

155. Tingling and numbness in the extremities ____

156. Inability to hold chiropractic adjustments ____

157. Watery eyes ____

158. Blurred vision ____

159. Productive cough, with yellow-green mucus ____

160. Chronic sinusitis ____

161. Wheezing ____

162. Nocturnal sweats ____

163. Bizarre dreams ____

164. Early morning fatigue ____

165. Attacks of faintness ____

166. Attacks of anxiety ____

HOW TO SCORE YOUR ANSWERS

Triggering Factors Section:

Questions 1 - 9: <u>10 points for each yes answer.</u>
Questions 10 - 24: <u>5 points for each yes answer.</u>
Question 25: <u>25 points for a yes answer.</u>
Question 26: <u>20 points for a yes answer.</u>
Questions 27 - 29: <u>15 points for each yes answer.</u>
Questions 30 - 32: <u>12 points for each yes answer.</u>

Questions 33 - 35: <u>10 points for each yes answer.</u>

Questions 36, 37: <u>8 points for each yes answer.</u>

Questions 38, 39: <u>5 points for each yes answer</u>.

Question 40: <u>15 points for a yes answer.</u>

Question 41: <u>10 points for a yes answer.</u>

Question 42: <u>20 points for a yes answer</u>.

Questions 43, 44: <u>15 points for each yes answer.</u>

Question 45: <u>12 points for a yes answer.</u>

Questions 46 - 57: <u>10 points for each yes answer.</u>

Question 58: <u>8 points for a yes answer.</u>

Question 59: <u>5 points for a yes answer.</u>

Questions 60 - 62: <u>15 points for each yes answer</u>.

Question 63: <u>10 points for a yes answer.</u>

Question 64: <u>15 points for a yes answer.</u>

Questions 65, 66: <u>10 points for each yes answer.</u>

Question 67: <u>8 points for a yes answer.</u>

Questions 68 - 70: <u>5 points for each yes answer.</u>

Question 71: <u>10 points for a yes answer.</u>

Questions 72 - 87: <u>5 points for each yes answer</u>.

Question 88: <u>10 points for a yes answer.</u>

Question 89: <u>5 points for a yes answer</u>.

Questions 90 - 107: <u>5 points for each yes answer.</u>

Total Section A Score: _____

Symptoms Section:

Questions 108 - 166

Never (N)	0 points
Occasional (O)	2 points
Moderate (M)	4 points
Severe (S)	6 points

Total Section B Score: _____

Now add totals from Sections A and B:

Your Final Score: _____

If you scored between 0 and 150, congratulations! You have been taking care of your immune system, most likely through an excellent lifestyle. It is very unlikely that you have any of the immuno-suppressed conditions present. But don't stop there! By following the Peak Immunity diet, covered in Chapter Eleven, you can make sure your immune system stays strong and defended against illness.

If your score is between 150 and 300, you are moving towards calamity — too many triggering factors most probably have already weakened your immune system. It is time to make lifestyle changes, because you might already be suffering from one or more immuno-suppressed conditions. Chapters Four through Eight, on various viral, yeast and parasitic conditions, can be helpful. You'll be able to get the help you need.

If your score is between 300 and 600, there is a very great chance that you suffer from one or more immuno-suppressed conditions. Consult your doctor immediately and ask for the appropriate test as explained in Chapters Four through Eight. Lifestyle changes are imperative!

If your score is between 600 and 1,200, filling out this questionnaire brought you no news; you know you are not doing well, to say the least. What you might not have known is that you are suffering from an immuno-suppressed condition. Seeking help from your physician is critical.

Whatever your score, turn to the next chapter to find out more about the various triggering factors threatening your health.

CHAPTER TWO

WHAT CAN TRIGGER ILLNESS?

You have just taken the self-scoring questionnaire. You may be curious about some of the questions you were asked. For instance, how would cooking with aluminum pots and pans affect your immune system?

Chronic Fatigue and Immune System Dysfunction Syndrome (CFIDS) is not caused by a single virus. Rather, it is the end result of years of subjecting the immune system to stress. In the case of aluminum cooking ware, that metal causes a build-up of toxins in the liver, causing it to function at a lower level. The accumulation of aluminum in the body is also a suspected factor in causing Alzheimer's disease. To improve your health and your immune system, you must be aware of such factors. This chapter will help you examine your lifestyle and environment, and determine what you can change for the better.

Stress factors take many forms. Some of the factors you cannot help. Your heredity, for instance, cannot be changed. If someone in your family has diabetes, that increases your risk of developing the disease. But there are many other factors within your control. This book has been designed to help you recognize contributing factors and to get help changing them.

Many physicians, because they have been trained in the Western tradition, tend to see illness as an isolated phenomenon. As a result, researchers have tried to find a single virus which is responsible for CFIDS. However, when physicians are able to see their patients as *whole human beings*, many other factors come into play which can help with the diagnosis.

The ancient practice of acupuncture, developed by the Chinese some 5,000 years ago, takes into account the person's entire being, physical and emotional, as well as exterior factors, in treating disease. For the Chinese, it was simple: nature and mankind cause disease, and nature has the cure for it. By understanding the triggering factors of your condition, you can find the way, through natural healing methods, back to peak immunity.

In the self-scoring questionnaire, you were asked about the triggering factors which might be present in your life. These factors come from the Chinese practice of medicine. The Chinese believed that the causes of disease can be divided into four main groups: hereditary factors, emotions, food (or nutrition) and external factors. Each of these factors could put a strain on the organs, which, according to the Chinese, had several well-defined functions. The Chinese saw the spleen and pancreas as a unified organ. Because of its role in the transportation and transformation of food, the spleen-pancreas plays a critical role in a healthy immune system. When this organ functions at a low level, malnutrition and underabsorption of nutrients can be the result. White blood cells, key defenders of the immune system, are produced in the spleen, as well as in the bone marrow and thymus. So if the spleen-pancreas is under-functioning, it's easy to see how the entire immune system, and its ability to fight off disease, would be affected.

In this chapter, we will explore the role of each of the four factors in causing disease.

1. Hereditary Factors

We cannot change our heredity — at least, not yet. Various diseases are passed from parents to their children. Some, like Tay-Sachs disease, are life-threatening. Others are not, but pose a lifelong sentence of chronic illness (such as with diabetes), or the development of rheumatoid arthritis. However, you don't need to feel helpless in the face of hereditary disease. If you know that the incidence of diabetes runs high in your family, you can take steps to control the three other factors (food, emotions and external factors) to help avoid, or, at least, diminish the intensity of the disease for yourself.

What this means is that hereditary diseases of the spleen-pancreas, such as diabetes, certain purpura or bleeding diseases and hypoglycemia, affect the strength of the immune system more than is generally thought. In simple terms, someone with diabetes already has a compromised immune system. Thus, they're more at risk for developing CFIDS.

Another common condition found in a family history is low thyroid function. This will lead to a decreased metabolism with maldigestion and malabsorption of nutrients. The digestive organs will be stressed, and the pancreas is one of them. The additional stress to your digestive system can lead to a compromised immune system. When CFIDS patients exhibit thyroid antibodies in their blood tests, this indicates the need for thyroid replacement therapy.

2. Emotional Factors

The second and third sections of the questionnaire dealt with your personality and with stressful life events. Eastern medicine has long recognized that the health of your psyche is important to your overall general health. (And, in fact, with psychoanalysis, Western medicine began to look at how emotional imbalance affected a person's physical health too.)

The Chinese believed that disease can start with a psychological disturbance. They concentrated on seven emotional factors: anger, joy, pensiveness, grief, melancholy, worry and fear.

When these emotions are in balance, there is no psychological disorder. In fact, even a healthy person needs to express each of these emotions to a certain degree. Only then are you well balanced. For instance, fear is the appropriate response when you encounter a dangerous situation. On the other hand, too much sustained fear can immobilize you, leaving you helpless and unable to react when situations demand action. Fear causes a chemical reaction in the body, whereby the adrenal glands secrete more adrenaline, stimulating the body to speed up the automatic responses. If these chemicals circulate in the blood for too long a period without a discharge, they begin to stress the organs, especially the adrenal cortex.

Each emotion in the Chinese model was linked to a specific organ. This relationship had radical consequences. Too much of a particular emotion can damage the correlated organ. And once that emotion decreases the energy in the corresponding organ, the weakness in this organ will lead to an increase of the emotion itself. For instance, fear, according to the Chinese, leads to a decrease in the energy for the kidney. When the kidney becomes weaker, patients with this condition will experience even more fear, completing the vicious cycle.

Often an organ operating at decreased capacity is not picked up by Western laboratory tests which may not be sensitive enough. In that case, the physician would look at the patient's clinical symptoms. In the case of a lack of energy in the kidneys, the patient would notice back pains, frequent urination, indecisiveness, migrating joint pains, ringing in the ears and hair loss. When properly noted, these symptoms can play a role in the early diagnosis of rheumatoid arthritis.

The Damage from Competitiveness

The questionnaire asked you several questions about hostility and competition. These hook into the importance the Chinese placed on worry or stress and anger.

Western medicine has made much of the type-A personality and its link to disease. Too much worry or stress, emanating from a compulsive, driven personality, can make a person particularly vulnerable to immune-suppressed diseases.

People with type-A personalities are excessively competitive and seem to experience constant time pressure. Every task has a sense of urgency about it. As a result, these people often have no patience with others. Type-A people may easily become hostile, are aggressive and extroverted, usually dominating in conversations and social gatherings. Do you recognize yourself? If so, you may be well on your way to a suppressed immune system! For you, the key to peak immunity may lie in finding ways to relax on a regular basis.

Worry and Anger

Anger, and its link to the liver, was also a critical emotion in the Chinese view. Too much anger can hamper the liver's ability to detoxify the blood, leading to stomach and liver pain and increased irritability and frustration, thus beginning the cycle all over again.

So worry and anger are the two main emotions linked to the suppression of the immune system. There is no doubt that these stress factors are the major triggering factors causing development of CFIDS. Often an emotional trauma or stressful event will be the final blow dealt to an immune system that was, perhaps, already weakened by unhealthy food intake, overprescribed antibiotics and other medications, and a stressful and polluted environment.

Unfortunately, because of the emotional content of these triggering factors, physicians are inclined to diagnose the patient as simply "being depressed." In the next sections, you will find out about the various tests which can be done to screen for the physical conditions which are responsible for making you ill.

3. Nutritional Factors

Although the old saying, "you are what you eat" has been with us for a long time, we don't really believe this as thoroughly as did the Chinese. Although it's common knowledge that your body needs proper nutrition to function properly, there is little agreement about what constitutes proper nutrition in this country.

The Chinese believed that the taste of food was important in keeping organs in balance. If a person takes in too much or too little of a certain taste, the corresponding organ's energy decreases. The taste associated with the spleen-pancreas, and thus important to the immune system, is the sweet taste.

Americans consume over 15 times the amount of sugar that they did 100 years ago. Excessive sugar intake has been linked to arthritis, hypertension, diabetes, dental decay and, equally important, depression and fatigue.

In our efforts to cut down on sugars, we have turned to non-caloric sweeteners. Picking up on Americans' preoccupation with weight loss, smart businessmen introduced saccharin in the 1960's and, in early 1981, another zero-calorie sweetener, Nutrasweet ™, made from aspartame, was given the go-ahead by the federal Food and Drug Administration (FDA).

The consequences of these noncaloric sweeteners have been disastrous. Nutrasweet ™, for instance, is about 200 times sweeter tasting than a comparable amount of white sugar. So by introducing saccharin and Nutrasweet ™ into your body, you decrease the amount of energy in the spleen-pancreas, and the immune system is depressed.

These sweeteners do nothing to induce permanent weight loss. As you can already guess, the ability of the spleen-pancreas to transform foods will be hampered by the excessive quantity of sweet taste. In other words, it is possible for the digestive capacities to decrease each time you ingest aspartame. The final result could be weight gain.

CFIDS sufferers often share a craving for sweets. Indulging the craving, however, only serves to further aggravate their symptoms. Chapter Eleven will give you tips on how to combat those cravings, and tells you which sweeteners (only the most natural) will be safe to use. You do not need to cut out sweets altogether. After all, the sweet taste is one of the necessary ones. But you do need to keep in mind that all sweeteners are concentrated simple sugars. So they cannot be considered whole foods. If you eat whole foods, their vitamins, minerals, and enzymes will allow smooth metabolism of the sugars that are within them.

The Chinese also believed that the environment (exterior and interior) was important to the proper functioning of the organs and the immune system. Cold-dampness and heat-dampness were the two properties damaging the spleen-pancreas. Raw, cold foods, the Chinese believed, which transform in the spleen to heat-dampness, slow down the organ's transforming capacities.

Our Food - Is It Safe?

Not only do most Americans eat improperly, adding too many processed foods and sweets to their daily intake, the so-called healthy foods may pose additional risks of their own. One of the prime examples of this is the routine addition of antibiotics to feed chickens, cows, and pigs. Livestock growers maintain that this is necessary to prevent bacterial infection in animals raised for food. However, these antibiotics may also induce the production of other bacteria resistant to them, leading to even more contamination of our meat and poultry supply.

Government studies indicate that 14% of dressed meat and poultry sold in supermarkets may contain illegal residues of drugs, pesticides or contaminants. Chapter Thirteen provides you a partial list of the most harmful additives, and supplies you with ways to avoid ingesting them.

Fat Content of Your Foods

By now, almost everyone has heard the American Heart Association's advisories about limiting fat intake. Ingesting too many fatty foods can lead to atherosclerosis, a disease in which fatty deposits build up on the artery walls, eventually leading to heart attack and stroke because of restricted blood flow. Also, fatty foods are more difficult to digest, thus hampering the functioning of the spleen-pancreas. The Brigham and Women's Clinic in Boston directed a study, which was published in the December, 1990, issue of *The New England Journal of Medicine*. That study found that the more red meat and fat people ate, the more likely they were to develop colon cancer. The researchers found that the women who ate red meat as a main course every day were two and a half times more likely to develop colon cancer than the women who ate meat sparingly or not at all. Eating chicken and fish, according to the study, did not contribute to the risk of colon cancer.

4. Exterior Factors

Sensitivity to Climate

You may be more sensitive to weather changes than other people. This is nothing new to the Chinese, who believed that the climate factor was one of the most important elements in the origin of disease. They believed that exterior-dampness, either hot or cold, was the most damaging climate to the immune system, since it decreases the strength of the spleen-pancreas organ, by stagnating and decreasing its energy. Following this line of thinking, living in the deep South, the Caribbean, or the Pacific Northwest is not a good idea for CFIDS sufferers. The reason? These areas get a lot of rain. Areas like the Southwest - Arizona, New Mexico - and the mountain areas, because the air is less humid, seem to be less damaging to the spleen-pancreas. On the other hand, someone with lung disease or asthma may not thrive in a dry climate, and may need more exterior moisture to be healthy.

The sudden appearance of a hot, dry wind (the Santa Ana in California, the chinook in the Rocky Mountain states, the *foehn* in Germany and the *sharav* in the Middle East) can trigger not only an aggravation of all CFIDS symptoms, but also depression and other alterations in behavior. The reason? These winds alter the chemistry of common environmental gases, such as nitrogen, oxygen and hydrogen, upsetting the balance in various brain transmitters such as serotonin, dopamine and norepinephrine. So the next time you feel depressed and see a sudden change in your CFIDS symptoms, take a look at the weather. A temporary aggravation may be nothing more than "weather madness."

Besides the climate factor, other exterior factors are equally important. These are factors that the Chinese, 5,000 years ago, never dreamed of:

Pesticides in the soil and air: After World War II, the agriculture industry used pesticides, such as DDT, to increase production on farm lands. Although DDT is now outlawed, other pesticides and artificial fertilizers are still in use. Chapter Thirteen provides tips on how to avoid ingestion of pesticides, where to shop for food that is safely grown, and techniques for preparing your food in the safest way possible.

Environmental irritants: One of the greatest dangers of pollution may well be that the human body is able to tolerate levels too low to cause awareness, but sufficiently high, nevertheless, to cause delayed pathological effects and to downgrade the quality of life. For instance, smog has not only a cumulative effect, causing disease at some time in the future, it constitutes a problem of continuing illness as well. The carbon monoxide hampers the ability to take in oxygen, affecting the brain function and contributing to the "brain fog" of the CFIDS patient. Because loss of short-term memory, headaches and fatigue are common health problems, their cause is not directly obvious and is often missed.

What is not known about air pollution may be even more distressing. Thousands of commercial compounds enter your environment each year. Some are proven cancer-causing substances, and many more are suspected of being so. The word "aerial soup" is well chosen; rarely do you suffer from just one or two air pollutants.

At the beginning of 1987, in the Public Health Service's annual report, U.S. Surgeon-General C. Everett Koop warned that so-called "involuntary" smoking — simply breathing in the vicinity of people with lighted cigarettes in enclosed areas — can cause lung cancer and other illnesses in otherwise healthy nonsmokers.

Pollution of our water supplies: The EPA reports that gases and compounds are leaking into underground water supplies from garbage dumps and landfills. The agency further states that 45% of large public water systems served by ground water are contaminated by organic and inorganic chemicals. There is still plenty of water on earth, but the problem is that more of it has been made undrinkable — by nature and by man.

Overuse of medications: In our result-oriented culture, the biggest premium is put on "results," and most patients are impatient with "process." The development of the "magic bullet" has gained prominence with the advances in cancer treatments, eradication of infections, and in the control of many common neuroses and psychological disorders. But addiction to prescription medication is perhaps one of the most insidious conditions of modern society.

Also, there are commonly used drugs, which may, rather than making the immune system stronger, weaken it, leaving it vulnerable to disease. Antibiotics such as penicillin, tetracyclines, sulfamides and the more modern cephalosporins (Cepro, Suprax) kill not only bacteria, but also your healthy flora, leading to yeast overgrowth and systemic infection. The dangers of cortisone loom over the patient, almost entirely cancelling its advantages. Systematic corticosteroid therapy causes Cushing's, diabetes, stomach ulcers and bleeding; it masks infections, delays wound healing and above all, it causes a fluctuation in the number of defender white blood cells, which exerts an immunosuppressive effect that increases the risk of Candidiasis, an important disease organism in CFIDS patients.

Many drugs available over-the-counter, such as indomethacin (Brufen ™), and the accepted chemotherapeutic agents for cancer therapy, have one thing in common: they can suppress white blood cells, leaving the door wide open to viruses, bacteria and yeast cells.

Life-style changes: The extraordinary life-style changes that occurred in the 60's are partly to blame for the immuno-suppressed conditions today. The 60s brought such drugs as marijuana, cocaine, LSD, and heroin into the mainstream. All these drugs disrupt the natural balance of the internal organs, especially the liver and spleen-pancreas. The 60s was also a time of sexual experimentation, increasing the incidence of sexually-transmitted diseases such as gonorrhea, syphilis and especially herpes simplex 2, or genital herpes. All these infections, either because of intake of antibiotics or because of the latent presence of the virus, decreased the strength of the immune system, making people more susceptible to the recent surge of CFIDS and other immune-suppressed diseases like AIDS.

Other Toxic Substances:

* Mercury dental fillings: In December 1990, 60 *Minutes,* CBS' nationally televised feature program, aired an excellent survey of the filling controversy. The American Dental Association is adamant that mercury fillings are non-toxic and completely safe. However, many countries in Europe (Sweden, Germany) have banned the use of mercury after clinical reports indicated that mercury fillings are toxic and may lead to brain degeneration.

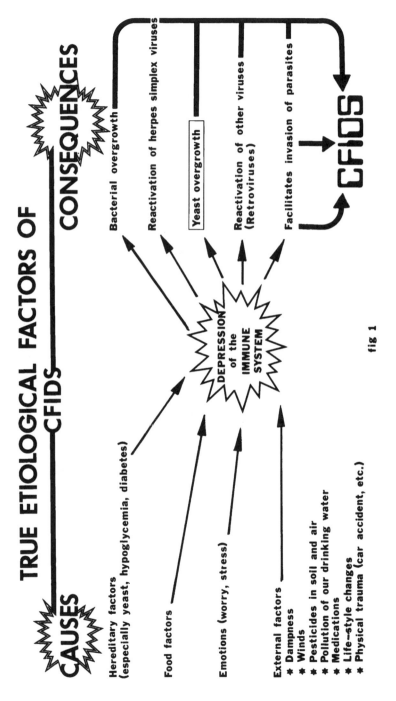

fig 1

On the left appear various co-factors, which, if present in sufficient numbers, will weaken the immune system, leaving it vulnerable to a variety of immune-suppressed conditions, and finally CFIDS.

Still, many questions remain unanswered. How can you know in advance whether removal of your mercury fillings will benefit you? You can't. Because it is a sensitivity (a broad term involving allergic, immunological, biochemical and biological reactivity) and not an allergy (a specific mechanism involving immediate or delayed hypersensitivity) to mercury that is the problem. The patients most likely to benefit from removal are the CFIDS patients loaded with food and environmental sensitivities. Patients who have tried everything else might be wise to replace their mercury fillings with for instance, inorganic cement (such as "Fleck's Zinc Cement" manufactured by the Mizzy Co.). Ask your dentist to recommend a course of action for you.

* Breast implants: Another program aired in 1990 by CBS tackled the problems experienced by patients with breast implants. Since 1960, some two million women have had breast implants. The procedure involves surgical placement of a device with an outer shell of silicone and silicone gel on the inside. Many women with breast implants have experienced leakage from these devices. Some silicone implants are covered with polyurethane foam (called "Meme" or "Replicon"). This foam can possibly peel away from the surface and spread all over the chest wall. There are no statistics on how many women have become ill because of their breast implants. Sensitivity to silicone may be documented through a blood test, such as those conducted by Dr. Kossovsky, of the University of California in Los Angeles, Department of Pathology.

Citing a series of concerns about breast implants (hardening of surrounding breast tissue, silicone leaks, false-positive mammogram readings and breast infections), the FDA gave the makers of silicone breast implants 90 days from April, 1991, to prove that these devices are safe. The latest findings by FDA researchers determined that the implant coating (a polyurethane foam) can dissolve slowly in the body, creating a chemical found to cause cancer in laboratory animals. Of course, the manufacturer's own tests found that this dissolution was minimal. At this point, women are better off waiting for the recommendations of the FDA, due to come out in mid summer, 1991. Stay tuned.

As Figure 1 illustrates, a multitude of triggering factors can suppress the immune system, leading to CFIDS. In the following chapter, you'll see how a healthy immune system combats intrusion from contaminants and disease.

CHAPTER THREE

YOUR BODY'S DEFENSES AGAINST ILLNESS

When treated with respect and care, your immune system takes care of your health 24 hours a day. In the state of peak immunity, your body is capable of resisting the invasion of viruses, parasites, yeast and bacteria.

We now know a great deal more about the immune system than we did 50 years ago. Modern medicine has made a major contribution to immunology through the discovery of powerful new laboratory methods.

However, when it comes to achieving "peak immunity" or "wellness," modern Western medicine doesn't provide the whole picture. Contemporary medicine is often "crisis management" medicine, rather than preventive medicine. Wellness is not only being symptom free, but also a state of inner peace that will balance the body. Wellness also means that you have control over your environment.

With the help of the diagrams on pages 32 to 38, this chapter outlines how your immune system works.

A Perfect Democracy

Every second of every day, battles rage within your body. Most of the time, you don't have the slightest idea about the incessant wars against invaders which are too tiny to see. A miracle of evolution, your body's immune system is an example of a perfect democracy, in which each member performs its particular task without being controlled by a superior central organ. The immune system provides the body with a 24-hour-a-day security system, always on the alert for viruses, harmful bacteria, fungi, protozoa, pollens and even malignant cells.

Like the specialized modern army, each type of cell has its own specific function. There are the combat troops (the phagocytes), capable of neutralizing the nearly invisible invaders. And there are the communications experts (T and B cells), which can accurately mark each target for the soldiers to destroy.

The core defenders are white cells, produced in the bone marrow and spleen, and divided into three groups. One kind are the phagocytes (so-called because they "eat" the invaders), the immune system's housekeepers. Then there are two types of lymphocytes ("cells in blood"), called T and B cells. All share one common objective: recognize and destroy all foreign bodies. These highly specialized white blood cells, about one trillion strong, engage in millions of battle encounters against formidable opponents. These are the "Star Wars" of your body.

The Battle Begins

Following is a description of how your immune system wages a typical battle against the simplest and yet most devious enemy: the virus. Consult the diagrams on pages 32 and 33 for a "cast of characters." It begins with the invasion. A virus such as the common cold virus is spread from one person to another through droplet infection. Someone sneezes on you, or you kiss someone, and if your immune system is not up to par, the virus, in its droplet carrier, enters your respiratory system. It follows the branches of the respiratory system into the smaller alveoli (small pouches in the lungs where oxygen exchange occurs) and gets absorbed into the smaller blood vessels. And in no time the battle has begun! How long it takes to have symptoms, or to defeat the virus entirely, depends on the strength of each person's immune system.

The first defenders to arrive are the phagocytes, the house cleaners of the system. Constantly alert, they roam through our bodies in the bloodstream, searching for anything that seems to be out of place. They waste no time — any invader they find is engulfed and consumed within seconds.

A special kind of phagocyte is the macrophage (or "big eater"), which literally eats the enemy, digesting and metabolizing its materials. Macrophages and other phagocytes are produced in the bone marrow and are present throughout the bloodstream and tissues of the body. Phagocytes are especially abundant in the liver, the organ responsible for filtering out toxins from the blood, and in the lungs, where they cleanse the tissue of airborne pathogens and particles. When the macrophage (the "Pac Man" of the immune system) attacks a virus, it plucks a special piece, called an antigen, located on the surface of the viral cell, from the invader. This antigen is then displayed on the surface of the macrophage like a captured war trophy. That trophy plays a critical role in the response of the fine machinery of the immune system. It will alert a highly classified kind of cell, the helper T-cell, commander-in-chief of our immune system.

Trained in the thymus gland, helper T-cells circulate throughout the bloodstream. These cells are so specific that there is only one that can read the antigen displayed on that macrophage and bind to it. In view of the hundreds of millions of antigens created by nature, the thymus confronts a staggering task, because it must turn out T-cells that recognize each enemy. But on with the battle plan! As we have seen, the T-cell binds to the macrophage through the displayed antigen and thus becomes activated. Once activated, helper T-cells begin to multiply. Like the battlefield general, their task is to send urgent chemical signals to a smaller squadron of soldiers—the killer T-cells, also trained to recognize one specific antigen. Once they receive the message from the helper T-cells, this little squadron multiplies into an irresistible army. They either puncture the cell membranes of bacteria with chemical secretions or destroy infected cells before the virus has time to multiply. Because the inside of the cell is the only place where the virus can replicate, the viral replication cycle is disrupted right there.

Helper T-cells also rush towards the spleen and lymph nodes to call on a second platoon of well-trained soldiers, the B-cells. These cells are produced in the bone marrow and migrate primarily to our lymph nodes. We only become aware of these bean-shaped capsules during infections, when they become swollen and sometimes painful to the touch, a sign that the immune system is fighting back. The lymph nodes are widely distributed throughout the body and are normally less than one-half inch long. These lymph nodes are strategically placed at crossroads, which might be compared to the way an army commander places his troops at mountain passes. During infections, B-cell lymphocytes trap the invaders in the lymph nodes, removing them from the bloodstream.

CAST OF CHARACTERS

 A virus is the cause of most common diseases. It is the simplest, yet the most devious enemy.

 A Macrophage, the body's "Pac Man" roams throughout our body, consumes pollutants and other invaders at a restless rate.

 The T-Helper cell, the commander-in-chief of our immune system. The fine mechanism of our defense system depends on its ability to activate the other defender-cells.

 The T-Killer cell, activated by the T-Helper cell, has only one goal: destroy the enemy before it has time to multiply.

 The B-cell, activated again by the T-Helper cell multiplies in the spleen and lymph nodes. They produce their weapons called antibodies.

fig 2

These are the "cast of characters" for the battles fought by your immune system.

CAST OF CHARACTERS CONT.

 Antibodies, produced by B-cells, stick to the surface of viruses, slow them down, but are also able to kill viruses.

 T-Suppressor cell will call the battle off when victory has been achieved. They tell the T-Killer cells to stop the fight.

 T-Memory cell stays in the body after the infection. It is trained to recognize the invasion of the same enemy in the future.

 B-Memory cell has the same function as the T-Memory cell. It will produce antibodies, upon recognizing the same enemy.

fig 2 cont.

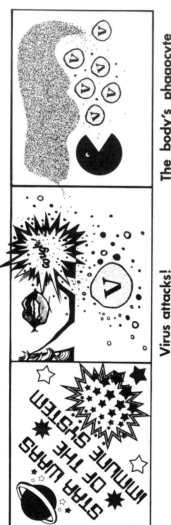

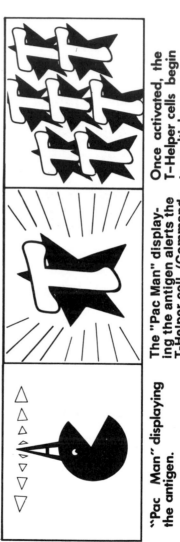

fig 3

The Star Wars of the Immune System: How your body's defenses react to invasion by a virus.

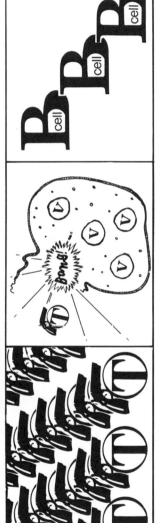

Like a battlefield general, the T-Helper cells send for the front soldiers called T-Killer cells!

They puncture membranes of the infected cells, disrupting the cycle of the viruses.

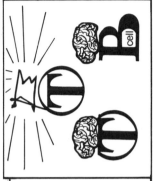

The T-Helper cells then call in the second platoon called B-Cells!

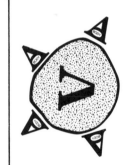

The B-Cells produce chemical weapons called antibodies.

Antibodies not only neutralize, but kill.

A truce is signed by the T-Suppressor. T and B-Memory cells are left in our body.

fig 3 cont.

The B-cells function as small munitions factories, producing chemical weapons called antibodies. When the killer T-cells puncture the membranes of the infected cells, the virus spills out where antibodies of the B-cells can directly bind to the surface of the virus, preventing it from killing other cells. By sticking to the surface, these antibody molecules slow down the virus enough to make it an easier target — as well as a more attractive one — for phagocytes. Antibodies do not only neutralize; they also kill! They fit on the enemy's antigen like a key in a lock and collect substances in the bloodstream, called complement. The latter can detonate like a bomb, destroying the invader's cell membrane. The reproductivity of these B-cells is truly amazing: at the peak of their operation, they can turn out thousands of antibodies a second, creating an awesome army.

By this time, you are experiencing the classic "cold" symptoms — runny nose, sore throat, congestion and overall "blahs."

Considering the size and sophistication of the body's armies, it is no small wonder that we win millions of battles. As the tide of these battles turns and the invaders are in retreat, a third member of the T-cell group takes command. These are the suppressor T-cells, and they are ready to sign a truce by releasing substances that turn off B-cells and other T-cells. They order them to stop fighting: the battle is won. You can imagine the debacle that would result if we did not have enough of these suppressor T-cells: the killer T and helper T-cells would continue to multiply out of control, resulting in the eventual exhaustion of the immune system.

The Battle Is Over

In the aftermath of these immune system wars, the army of housecleaners empties the battlefields of the litter of dead cells. The battles are over, but not forgotten by the immune system. Most of the T and B-cells will die off within days. But a large contingent will lead long lives and roam through the body as so-called memory cells. They will enable the body to respond more quickly to subsequent infections. If and when we encounter the same enemy, the battle will be over in a matter of seconds. The virus is recognized immediately and overwhelmed by the right kind of antibodies. In other words, you are immune to that particular virus.

This is the way your immune system functions when it is well and getting the proper fuel from good nutrition and a nonpolluted environment.

Something Goes Wrong

If everything ran as smoothly as described above, you would be in good shape. Unfortunately, your T-cells are so diligent that they recognize even what are considered desirable cells, transplanted from one person to another, identify them as foreign and destroy them. This process, called rejection, can defeat a life-saving heart or kidney transplant and put a patient back to ground zero.

Even more problematic is a category of illnesses called autoimmune diseases, in which the immune system attacks its own cells because it mistakenly takes them for foreign bodies. Examples of these diseases are rheumatoid arthritis, a disease of the joints, systemic lupus erythematosus (with skin and kidney involvement), Crohn's disease (a bowel disorder), ulcerative colitis (a disease of the bowels), and scleroderma, with changes primarily in skin and circulation.

At this point in time, medicine does not have a remedy for these diseases. Using the drug cortisone will suppress the activity of the immune system, so that the body does not attack itself. This also means, however, that the body's resistance to infection is decreased. So, for instance, a kidney transplant patient who must take cortisone to curb rejection of the transplant is also much more susceptible to the common cold — and its complications can become life-threatening.

As medical students, my peers and I called cortisone "the blessing of a false bishop." That's because cortisone gives people an initial euphoric action, which makes them feel very energetic and powerful. But with prolonged use, terrible side effects can occur, such as ulcers, osteoporosis, decreased resistance to infection, diabetes and Cushing's disease, to name just a few.

Rejection of a necessary transplanted organ is not the only error of judgment that the immune system makes. It sometimes mounts battles against phantom enemies. Thousands of harmless substances, such as pollen and dust, cause allergic reactions in some 40 million Americans. The allergen itself is no threat. Most people are exposed to it without any consequence. In hay-fever sufferers, however, the immune system mistakenly recognizes pollen as an enemy. The immediate reaction is a spill of potent chemicals, such as histamine, released by specialized mast cells. And our faithful T-cells make matters worse by ordering B-cells to produce more antibodies. (See Fig. #4) So sneezing spells, runny noses and teary eyes are simply signs of an overreactive immune system.

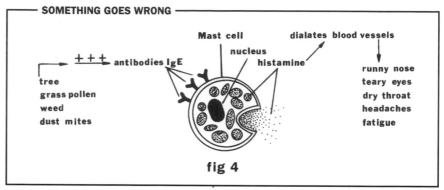

Something Goes Wrong: This drawing depicts what happens when your immune system over-responds, causing a release of histamine and resulting in the uncomfortable symptoms of allergy.

The System Goes On Overload

Often, CFIDS patients ask, "How can my immune system be weak? I have not gotten a single cold over the last year!" Using such an indicator of health creates a false sense of security. Analogous to the military camp, a small common cold virus has no chance to penetrate the immune system when it is functioning at high alert because it is fighting another yeast cell, bacteria or parasite continuously. But how long can this go on?

Keep a military camp on high alert for 24 hours a day and inevitably it will crack down. In the beginning, not one single enemy can penetrate this defense. Yet as days progress, the defenders in the camp get nervous. It is pure adrenaline that keeps them going, and wild, unwarranted shots are fired upon birds rustling in the trees. But no defense can hold up forever when it is involved in such a war.

Inevitably, white blood cells get killed in the continuing raging wars. You might be able to detect this in a regular blood panel reading showing that the number of white blood cells is just below the normal limit (3,700 for instance if the normal values are between 4,000 and 10,000). Such a white blood cell count could mean that the days of the healthy immune system are numbered. Before you know it, you are catching every cold that comes around; and a flu that keeps somebody else at home for one day keeps you in bed for a week. You may have the continuous presence of mucus, postnasal drip, sinusitis, cough, fatigue that is not alleviated by rest, and reactions towards cigarette smoke, car exhaustion and perfumes. Then you might experience an outbreak of herpes simplex I ("cold sores") or sexual herpes, after being free from them for over a decade.

Continuous sore throats, swollen glands and low grade fevers are other ominous signs that the immune system is breaking down. It is imperative for any patient who gradually experiences some of these symptoms, to view them for what they are: signs of a derailed immune system. Do not make the mistake of classifying them as separate symptoms, requiring some minor steps to rectify them. This is what happens to most CFIDS patients: symptomatic treatment with antibiotics can put them on the downhill trail toward poor health. It would be better to fortify your immune system by drastic changes in your lifestyle: improve your diet, start exercising and balance yourself emotionally. Do not, however, neglect to see your doctor when your symptoms warrant it. But you should also look to your diet and lifestyle for contributory factors.

You've seen in this chapter how the immune system functions to deflect and destroy microscopic invaders. Now, if you suspect that you may have CFIDS or be at risk for developing the syndrome, the next section should be especially helpful. In Chapter Four, the diagnostic tests for CFIDS are described in detail. This will help you as your doctor begins to make a diagnosis about your condition. Also included are several diseases which mimic CFIDS symptoms and which should be ruled out as possibilities. In Chapters Five through Eight, the related conditions of viral illness, yeast infections, parasitic involvement and AIDS will also be discussed. You'll also learn how to free yourself from symptoms that may have been troubling you for months, even years. When you are correctly diagnosed and treated for immuno-suppressed conditions, then you can start rebuilding your immune system. With proper diet, exercise and supplements, you can actually "boost" its capacity and regenerate your body's defenses.

SECTION TWO

JUST WHAT IS AILING YOU?
DESCRIPTIONS AND DIAGNOSIS
OF CFIDS AND OTHER MAJOR AILMENTS

CHAPTER FOUR

IS CFIDS YOUR DIAGNOSIS?

Janet, 40 years old, had suffered from food allergies from birth on. Growing up, she seemed to cope better with the "colic" and milk intolerance that were so much a part of her young life. But her health took a turn for the worse in adolescence, when she took tetracyclines for acne problems, followed by birth control pills to regulate her menstrual cycle. She remembered being chronically tired in high school, with a lack of concentration and poor short-term memory. Frequent colds and sore throats prompted doctors to prescribe antibiotics which at first seemed to make her feel better. But very quickly, she reacted adversely to most antibiotics.

These symptoms lasted into Janet's adult life, and she struggled to have enough energy to cope with work and friends. At one point, she tried to recuperate in Mexico, only to come down with two days of "traveler's diarrhea." The trip left her exhausted. When she presented herself in our clinic, Janet was already resigned to the fact that she would never have a "normal" life with a work schedule like "normal" people. However, after diagnosing her with CFIDS, with involvement of yeast overgrowth and Entamoeba Histolytica, a parasite, adequate treatment for those conditions provided Janet with more energy than she had ever hoped for.

You just took the test in Chapter One, and you found that you've scored pretty high. What do you do? The first thing is not to panic or despair. There is help, and a way back to health. But first you must consult your physician and get help with your diagnosis. Reading this chapter will help you ask the right kinds of questions and find out whether your physician is ordering the appropriate tests.

One of the frustrating things about CFIDS is its elusive quality. Its exact cause has evaded medical researchers, who at first wanted to find the culprit virus or bacteria. No longer the outsider in medical diagnoses, CFIDS is nevertheless still hard to pin down in diagnostic testing. In the following pages, step-by-step testing and diagnostic findings help you see how you can get a definitive diagnosis.

According to your symptoms, your doctor will decide on certain tests. Several may be needed to establish a diagnosis of CFIDS. See the Appendix for the complete list of possible CFIDS symptoms. Reading this chapter will help you ask for other tests, and allow you to understand the results your doctor obtains. Now that you have learned about so many aspects of your health, there is a need and desire to put it in practice. That is what this chapter is all about. It will enable you to go to your doctor and ask him or her to perform certain tests that both of you think might be necessary according to your symptoms. Once your correct diagnosis has been established by your physician, you can apply the different therapeutic techniques you have found in this book.

Diagnostic Tests and Their Interpretation

Once CFIDS was considered a "legitimate" disease by the medical community, the search for the definitive diagnostic test was on. As you already understand, it is foolish to think that only one diagnostic test will be necessary to make the diagnosis of CFIDS. While some of the present tests discussed in the different chapters, and in this one, might be redundant in a couple of years, they are still the best at this point to help us unravel the mystery of CFIDS. I will discuss, step-by-step, the different findings the patient and the doctor have to look for.

Blood Tests a Must

A complete blood panel is one of the first tests ordered by physicians whose patients present the broad-ranging symptoms of CFIDS (see the Appendix for a list of possible symptoms).

What will we see in case of CFIDS patients and why?

* In approximately 50-75% of the CFIDS patients you see a decrease of the total white blood cells. This is a remarkable finding. Depending on the reference rates of the lab, a normal number is in

the range of 4,000 to 11,000. In CFIDS patients there is usually a slight decrease in this number, something like 3,500-3,800.

Even if this decrease isn't shown, comparing present white blood cell counts with previous CBC's will show a diminishing trend. Why? As you learned in Chapter Three, the white blood cells are the soldiers of our immune system. Battles with viruses, yeast or parasites may rage for years in your body. And the longer the battle goes on, the more casualties (loss of white blood cells) you will have. A decreased number of white blood cells should be one of the first alarm signs. It is important for doctors to recognize this. All too many patients suffering from CFIDS heard the diagnosis of MS or leukemia, even AIDS, before CFIDS came into the picture.

* A second, nearly always consistent, finding is a *slight* decrease in the other cells: the red blood cells (RBC's) and platelets (less often). Often, the diagnosis of anemia is made, and the doctor might think this is the single cause of your CFIDS. However, this anemia is usually not serious (except in advanced cases) and correction of this anemia, although desirable, will not bring the expected relief to the patient.

Where does this anemia come from? Victims of CFIDS have malabsorption. Compounded with yeast infections, which are also common with CFIDS, these patients absorb less vitamin B_{12} through their stomachs and upper intestines. This causes a vitamin B_{12} deficiency, technically called "pernicious anemia," and not a true iron deficiency, or "ferriprive anemia." Therapy will be an increased intake of B_{12}, by taking oral tablets or receiving intramuscular injections twice a week.

* A third finding, less present than the two previous ones, is a slight increase in some of the liver function tests, mostly the Transaminases (SGPT/SGOT), which are the liver enzymes, measuring the detoxification function of the liver. Again, misunderstanding might lead to unnecessary liver biopsies or ultrasound of the liver (the latter at least less dangerous). Why this increase of liver enzymes? It is a clear sign that your liver is suffering. This is directly related to its most important function: the detoxification of the body. With CFIDS patients liver biopsies and ultrasound will turn out to be normal most of the time, and therefore should be less frequently performed upon finding minor changes in these liver enzymes.

If you suffer from CFIDS and one of your symptoms is chronic constipation, you can overwhelm the liver with toxin build up. This is sometimes very clear clinically: patients will have high stomach pain and later on, strong pains in the liver area. The increased liver enzymes are an alarm sign that your liver cannot fulfill its primary function, the cleansing of your body. How to deal with this is extensively discussed in Chapter Twelve. Other symptoms of liver "intoxication" are elevated blood cholesterol levels, and frequent bruising because the blood clotting factors are fabricated in the liver. (Frequent bruising is also a symptom of other serious illnesses, so be sure to get such a symptom checked out by your doctor.)

  * A very important part of this blood panel is the *thyroid panel*. However, the thyroid panel is probably one of the least sensitive tests available.

Temperature Monitoring

The Barnes Basal Temperature is more accurate than the thyroid portion of your blood panel. It is also easy to administer at home. On the night before the test, shake down an oral thermometer and leave it on your bedside table. After waking the next morning, having abstained from alcohol the night before, remain in bed and place the thermometer firmly in your armpit for 10 minutes. Do not take your temperature by mouth, as this is not a reflection of your basal metabolism. If your reading is lower than 97.8 — normal resting temperature — you are very likely hypothyroid. With CFIDS patients, it is very common to see temperatures below 97.0. Repeat the process the next morning. If you are a woman of child-bearing age, perform the test only on the second and third day of menstruation. The combined results of basal temperature and thyroid blood tests (T3, T4 and TSH) will allow the physician to determine the course of therapy. An appropriate small oral dose of Synthroid or Armoured thyroid (consult your doctor), has done miracles for many CFIDS patients. It is interesting to note that the synthetic synthroid (T4) is always released in the same doses in your body, while the more natural Armoured thyroid (T3 and T4) has a more irregular release. This fluctuating release will give you changing relief of your symptoms, but your doctor should be able to establish the right amount for you.

Specific Tests

Once you know how to look at this regular panel, more specific tests are required. The different tests to exclude different pathogenic organisms are explained in their respective chapters.

* For candida, the Candida Antibody test in Chapter Six.
* For parasites, the Purged Stool test in Chapter Seven.
* For Herpes Simplex Viruses: EBV/CMV panel (IgG, NA, VCA and IgM), and possible Herpes Simplex levels I and II in Chapter Five.
* For AIDS, the ELISA and the Western Blot tests in Chapter Eight.

Again, it is imperative to understand that these viruses are consequences, not causes. In that light, I fully agree with the excellent study, "Chronic Fatigue Syndrome and the Diagnostic Utility of Antibody to Epstein-Barr Virus Early Antigen." by the Mayo Clinic (1), which concluded that "antibody to EBV early antigen is not helpful in the clinical evaluation of patients with CFIDS." However, increased antibody levels in a EBV/CMV panel will indicate to the patient and doctor the hyperactivity and the stress that the immune system has to endure. And of course, it will become important in therapy. An HIV test will always be encouraged, most of the time to give the patient peace of mind, something they can use when fighting for health.

Immune Panel

This is the next step in testing for CFIDS. The immune panel consists of the total white blood cell (WBC) count, the total lymphocytes, the T4 or Helper T-cells, the T8 or Suppressor T-cells, the T4/T8 ratio, the total B-lymphocytes, and the Natural Killer cells (NK's).
   * WBC *count*:
This is already part of the complete blood panel and was discussed above. What this blood panel shows is a differentiation between all the different kinds of white blood cells. It makes sense that if we want to have a battery of tests linked to CFIDS, that these tests will be found in the different kinds of white blood cells.
   As stated before, depending on the reference rates of the lab, a normal number of WBC is in the range of 4,000 to 11,000 WBC/cu

mm. In other words, when you go below 4,000, it indicates a weakness in your immune system: you simply have too few soldiers to throw into the battle. On the other hand, an increase in WBC (more than 11,000) is a sign of infection, with an adequate response of your immune system.

* Total Lymphocytes:

These are the T-and B-cells, the cornerstones of your immune system. They normally make up a certain percentage (25-40%) of your total WBC. Again, a decrease in this percentage indicates a weakened immune system.

* T4 or Helper T-cells:

These are the generals of your immune system, calling upon the other cells (B-cells, Killer T-cells) to help fight the enemy. Normally they comprise between 35 to 55% of the total lymphocytes. If your figure is far below the 35%, it means that your immune system is compromised — you don't have enough Helper T-cells to call for help, hence the attacker (virus, yeast cell, bacteria), has more time to multiply and further weaken your resistance. An extreme example will be AIDS, where most of the Helper T-cells are knocked out since the AIDS virus has been able to slip into this cell. As a result, the Helper T-cells are not giving any messages to the rest of the troops.

On the other hand, a figure above 55% indicates an "overactive" or "hyperactive" immune system, where too many Helper T-cells are summoned to fight a troupe of enemies. If this continues, the number of Helper T-cells will become exhausted, leading to the exhaustion of the immune system.

* Suppressor T-cells or T8 cells:

These soldiers have to call the fight off when the battle is won; their normal figure is in the range of 20% to 37% of total lymphocytes; too few T8 cells will cause the battle to continue unnecessarily, again exhausting the number of T4 cells. Too many T8 cells will call the battle off prematurely, leaving the virus undefeated in your body.

* T4/T8 Ratio:

Ideally, you want 1.8 T4 cells for every T8 cell; in other words, the ratio will be roughly 1.8/1 or simply 1.8. If the ratio falls, you don't have enough T4 cells prodding the immune system into action.

* B-Cells:

These are "factories" where the antibodies are formed that slow down or neutralize the invaders. The normal amount is 5-25% of the total lymphocytes. Absence of, or a markedly reduced number of, B-cells is suggestive of immunodeficiency states. A marked increase is suggestive of malignancy states and helpful in the diagnosis of Chronic Lymphocytic Leukemia (CLL) and possible presence of an auto-immune disorder.

* Interleukin-2:

This is a glycoprotein released by the Helper T-cells. Functions of Interleukin-2 include T-cell proliferation, stimulation of interferon and B-cell growth factor, all very important in our defense system. The inability of the human T-cell to generate normal amounts of IL-2 is indicative of immunodeficiency seen in conditions such as AIDS, Candida, SLE (Systematic Lupus Erythematosus), Pemphigus and T-cell Leukemias.

The above findings are expressed in Table #1.

Typical Findings in a CFIDS Patient

* A decreased number of white blood cells
* An increase in T4 cells
* A T8 cell reading which is normal or slightly decreased
* A T4/T8 ratio above 1.8
* Usually, a decrease in the number of B cells, toward the lower border of normality. (If normal is between 5 and 20, the number will be close to or below 5.)
* A decrease in natural killer (NK) cell activity
* An increased cytokinine production (IL-2, or alpha interferon)
* An elevation of thyroid antibodies (indicative of Hashimoto's Disease), and antibodies to Herpes Simplex viruses, candida and Lyme disease.

All these abnormal levels (either increased or decreased) are an expression of the raging battles in your body, with your immune system in high alert and hyperactive, but suffering small defeats nevertheless. I have no doubt that in the near future, by focussing on these immune cells, scientists will be able to develop an immune panel that could be useful to confirm the diagnosis, and even more importantly, could gauge the effectiveness of drugs/supplements to treat CFIDS.

Cell Type	N1	Decreased	Increased
WBC	4,000-11,000	Too few defenders	Sign of infection
Lympho's	25-40% of WBC	Immune system down	Infection or cancer
T4	35-55% of Lympho's	The general of the immune system forgets to alert his troops	Overreactive immune system
T8	20-37% of Lympho's	Battles continues	Battle called off too early
T4/T8 Ratio	1.8	Suppressed immunity	Too many T4 or too few T8 cells
B-cells	5-25% of Lympho's	Not enough enemies neutralized	Overreactive immune system or cancer
Interleukin-2		Suppressed immunity	

table 1

Sorting Out Your Symptoms

In medicine there is something called a *differential diagnosis.* This means that the physician determines which disease you are suffering from by systematically comparing and contrasting the clinical findings. There are other diseases which can be confused with CFIDS. Due to the generality of the symptoms and the lack of adequate laboratory tests, doctors have a tendency to focus on certain symptoms of the patient in particular.

The following conditions can be confused with CFIDS. I present a brief description of each, so that patients who might hear these diagnoses from their physicians can urge them to do further testing to rule out these largely chronic diseases, which are either incurable or require a very extensive term of therapy with many side effects.

Multiple Sclerosis (M.S.); S.L.E. or Systemic Lupus Erythematosus; Interstitial Cystitis; Hypoglycemia; Fibromyositis or Fibromyalgia; Hypothyroidea, clinical depression and Lyme disease all show symptoms related to CFIDS. Unfortunately, there are plenty of people out there suffering from these conditions. However, it would be wise for the doctor and the patient to first rule out the diagnosis of CFIDS. Even if the diagnosis of these conditions is confirmed, patients can greatly benefit from the Candida/Peak Immunity diet (see Chapter Eleven). Let's have a closer look at these conditions.

Multiple Sclerosis

This condition hits at a young age, and a majority of victims are women between 30 and 45 years old. The disease may take one of two forms: either a relapsing, remitting disease of the nervous system (there is a degeneration of the myelin sheet around the nerves) or a chronic, progressive disease. Symptoms can be double vision, incontinence, fatigue, dizziness, and numbness and weakness in an extremity. The latter symptoms might be confused with CFIDS. There is no one single test that indicates with 100% certainty that one suffers from M.S. Rather, a battery of tests is performed: spinal tap, visual and auditory evoked potentials and MRI (magnetic resonance imaging) to show possible demyelinating plaques in the brain or spinal cord. There is no therapy for this condition, which is even more reason to explore every other possible diagnosis, CFIDS included. MRI's were taken during the first large outbreak of CFIDS in 1985 in Incline Village, Nevada. UBO's, or "unidentified bright objects" were noted in these patients' brains, increasing the possibility of confusion with M.S. (UBO's or demyelinated plaques are one of the prominent findings in patients with M.S.)

Systemic Lupus Erythematosus (SLE)

This is another autoimmune disease demonstrating an array of symptoms: depression, fatigue, kidney trouble and skin rashes, the most classical one being the "butterfly" rash — a rash in the form of a butterfly around the nose on both cheeks. It is frequently because of the presence of this rash alone that doctors start thinking about SLE. However, many candidiasis patients show this rash around the cheeks and nose. An ANA blood test should be performed, but I have seen this test become negative upon treating these patients for underlying factors such as candidiasis.

The therapy for SLE is cortisone. Not exactly what you would need if the diagnosis were really candidiasis.

Seborrheic eczema is another skin rash often due to candidiasis. This form of eczema is located mostly on the chest and head, where it is popularly known as dandruff. However, by culturing the white flakes for yeast, candida albicans often is isolated. The rash regresses when the patient follows an anti-yeast diet instead of again using cortisone creams.

Interstitial Cystitis

This is a rare disease for which no treatment is available. But its incidence is high enough to have warranted support groups of sufferers all over the country. Patients suffer from painful and frequent urination, possibly leading to a dysfunctional bladder if the situation persists. Urine cultures can be negative. A cystoscopy (where a lamp attached to a rod is unserted into the urethra to allow viewing inside the bladder) usually leads to a definitive diagnosis.

The cause of interstitial cystitis is unknown. The specialists treating these patients should also look for CFIDS, and especially the role played by candida and EBV. "Interstitial Cystitis" patients often test positive for candida and CEBV and frequently respond favorably to the anti-yeast diet and medication (see Chapter Nine). A possible reason for this is that because of the continuous irritation of the bladder mucosae, after years of releasing dead candida toxins via the bladder, the mucosa becomes irritated and will change subsequently to a 'rigid' nonfunctional bladder wall.

Hypoglycemia and Fibromyositis/Fibromyalgia

Hypoglycemia is nothing but a symptom taken out of the whole syndrome of CFIDS. Almost any CFIDS patient has been diagnosed at some point as being hypoglycemic. The patient can have crying spells, shakiness and weakness, with heart palpitations, and confusion if he or she goes too long between meals. Regular, more frequent small meals (protein, not sugar) will prevent these hypoglycemic swings. In a way, the diagnosis is not wrong but it is the same as considering fatigue a separate disease instead of being part of CFIDS.

The same is true for Fibromyositis or Fibromyalgia. As the name expresses, this name indicates inflammation and pain in the muscles and tendons. Especially in the neck, scapular and lower back area, the patient can experience severe muscle pains and spasms with buildup of muscle knots. Again, this is a constant symptom of CFIDS, not another disease. It is related to the buildup of toxins, released when the immune system kills viruses, parasites and yeast cells.

An excellent therapy for this condition is the intake of Magnesium: about 1,200 mg daily. Intake of this much Magnesium will also cause loose stools, but this is mostly desirable for CFIDS patients.

Depression

Up until 1990, many CFIDS patients were diagnosed as suffering from this "unbearable darkness of being." Scientists went as far as considering CFIDS patients just being depressed and nothing more. I think this is another example of how we confused the symptom with the cause. Who wouldn't be depressed if they were hit with a disabling disease that robbed them of any pleasure in life, that isolated them from their friends and family and created disbelief in their doctor?

When studies were done of CFIDS patients, they found that more of them were depressed than in a control group. But these patients often grew up in abusive or alcoholic families, putting a strain on their immune systems at an early age. But does this mean that CFIDS is equal to depression? This diagnosis is an insult to these unfortunate victims, not helpful for their self-esteem and strength to recuperate from this vicious condition.

This does not mean that depression in several forms does not exist. There is the chronic, less severe form of depression or dysthymia, with unrelenting lassitude and hopelessness, and postpartum depression, occurring in a certain percentage of women after giving birth.

Psychotherapists, psychiatrists and any other health practitioners should be acquainted with CFIDS and realize that besides psychological causes there will also be physical ones, to be corrected with other measures than just psychotherapy.

Lyme Disease

Lyme disease is an inflammatory disorder transmitted by the deer tick. The deer carry a spirochete (Borrelia) which can infect people and make them ill. Originally reported on the East coast, especially New Jersey, Lyme disease has now been found in at least 30 states, in forested areas as well as on suburban lawns.

The symptoms of Lyme disease can occur in three stages, either independently or overlapping.

* In the first stage, a "bull's eye" rash can appear on the limbs. However, this rash is present in only about 20% of the cases, and may go unnoticed by the patient. Additionally, and it is here that we can confuse CFIDS with Lyme's disease, patients can suffer from profound fatigue and flu-like symptoms such as fever, chills, muscle/joint aches and headaches.

* In a second stage, which may occur weeks or months after the tick bite, facial paralysis, short-term memory, numbness or pins and needle feelings in the limbs, meningitis (inflammation of the spinal cord), carpal tunnel syndrome (pain and stiffness in the wrist joints), extreme fatigue and heart pain (because of inflammation) may occur. Again, a lot of these symptoms can also be found in any CFIDS patient.

* Stage three, which sometimes occurs years after the bite, results in arthritis or persistent neurologic problems. But arthritic pains are not uncommon in CFIDS either.

The diagnosis of Lyme disease is a clinical one. There is no substitute for a detailed, in-depth history taken by the physician. None of the available tests is 100% accurate. Lyme serologies (Lyme antibody ELISA test, Western blot, the latter one difficult for the lab to interpret objectively) and T- and B-cell testing are helpful but by no means absolutely definitive. Spinal taps are not recommended, as a negative test will not rule out Lyme disease.

One can immediately see that it is difficult to make a difference clinically between CFIDS and Lyme's disease. Yet the consequences are disastrous. Imagine a patient who suffers from CFIDS with extreme yeast overgrowth and gets diagnosed with Lyme disease. The treatment for Lyme disease is antibiotics, sometimes intravenously, for several weeks to months. This continuous intake of antibiotics will favor the growth of yeast, which could be the real cause of the symptoms! The patient may feel worse, and the doctor may think, quite logically, that the antibiotic has not been given long enough or in high enough doses and may increase the time period and strength of the doses. This could become a real nightmare for the patient.

Besides performing the ITL candida antibody test described on pages 78-79, it would be better to first start a trial therapy with diet and antifungals, before taking any antibiotics. However, if there is a strong suspicion you may have Lyme disease (you were recently hiking in the woods, for instance, do not wait longer than 14 days to seek medical treatment. Lyme disease can become aggravated if proper treatment is delayed.

Treatment Guidelines for Lyme Disease

Because the Lyme spirochete distributes rapidly to all parts of the body, including the central nervous system, the chosen antibiotic must be able to penetrate all tissues in adequate concentration. Treatment may have to be continued for a long period of time to eradicate all symptoms and to prevent relapses. (The spirochete has a long generation period and may have periods of dormancy, only to flare up anew). Tetracyclines, such as doxycycline and minocycline, are somewhat effective in the early stages, but the effects are not lasting and relapses are common. The most effective antibiotics are the cephalosporins, such as ceftriaxone and cefiximine, but they are expensive and cause side effects such as nausea and vomiting.

Patients over the age of 60 seem to respond less well to antibiotics and may require intravenous therapy. This will necessitate getting complete blood counts and chemistry panels every six weeks to monitor any possible toxicity of the therapy. Anyone on this type of medication should avoid drinking alcohol or exposure to sunlight and should get proper rest.

* If you need long-term penicillin or cephalosporin therapy, you need to remember that this can lead to an overgrowth of yeast. To counteract the killing off of the normal flora in your body, take acidophilus at the same time. Just eating extra yogurt will not do the job.

The "Burning" Vagina

Most gynecologists are familiar with a condition in which patients complain of a burning vagina that is tender to the touch and is one of the major causes of painful sexual intercourse. This is sometimes referred to as vulvodynia, analogous to glossodynia or burning tongue.

The cause of this condition is still unknown. Several culprits have been suggested, among them human papillomavirus or HPV, which causes tumorous growths in the vagina, Trichomonas, a protozoa that causes infection, or Gardnerella, a major cause of bacterial vaginitis. If found, these infections are treated, but treatment does not always relieve the burning sensation.

Holistic doctors have noticed a close connection between the presence of candida albicans and the inflamed vagina. Again, we do not refer only to the local vaginal yeast infection, but to the widespread epidemic of the yeast hypersensitivity syndrome. Often, patients apply local creams to the vagina, which causes an aggravation of the burning. As you will see in the chapter on yeast infections, burning of the mucosae (anal, vaginal, bladder) and skin in general is very common. A possible explanation is that the body tends to get rid of dead candida cells, or toxins, through any possible opening in the body. This continuous release of toxins irritates the mucosae and leads to these complaints and sometimes permanent changes as seen in interstitial cystitis.

If these symptoms apply to you, the therapy for yeast infections would be an excellent one to follow. Outlined in Chapter Nine, the therapeutic measures include diet restrictions, anti-fungal medications or supplements and preferably a local, natural therapy to relief the discomfort. The latter can be chosen between local douching with liquid garlic, Pau D'Arco, Australian tea tree oil, acidophilus, (all 1 Tablespoon to 3 oz of water) or baking soda (1 tsp) in water. There are also natural suppositories available, one of them called EPC suppo's. They get the name from their ingredients: Echinacea, Pau D'Arco and Chapparal. Holistic doctors have seen considerable success in combatting this unfortunate condition with these methods.

One of the puzzles for medical doctors is the fact that repeated smears and vaginal cultures turn out negative for candida. No active infections could be found, which is understandable when you accept the above theory of toxin release: how could you culture something that is dead? Negative smears and cultures for yeast should not be a reason for not trying the above outlined anti-candida regime.

For further reading on this condition, which can sometimes be confused with other maladies, see the reference section at the end of the chapter.

Mitral Valve Prolapse (MVP)

* What Is MVP?

Mitral valve prolapse is a heart condition in which a leaky valve situated between the left forechamber (atrium) and chamber (ventricle), allows a back flow of blood from the ventricle into the atrium as the blood is being pumped to the rest of the body. (See Figure 5). It is a condition that can be discovered by your doctor, who hears a "click" sound when the condition is severe enough.

A diagnosis of MVP is confirmed by a test called an echocardiagram, a noninvasive ultrasound of the heart, which can give the technician a picture of the extent of the leak.

* Is It Risky?

There is still a debate about the seriousness of this condition in the medical world. MVP should not interfere with normal activities and life expectancy, but some cardiologists contend that it could be responsible for thousands of sudden deaths among the population. The biggest risk posed is of infection, especially during dental procedures and with congestive heart failure. As a preventative measure, MVP patients are given oral antibiotics before major dental procedures. Although nothing is proven, these people may be more prone to stroke and arrhythmia (irregularities in the heartbeat).

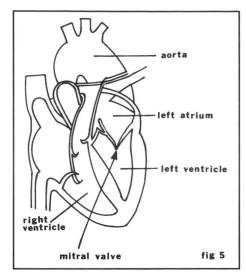

aorta

left atrium

left ventricle

right ventricle

mitral valve   fig 5

This cutaway drawing of the heart shows the location of the mitral valve, situated between the left atrium and left ventricle. If this valve does not close properly, it can cause leakage and let in infections which can be serious if precautions are not taken before dental and other procedures.

* Is It Common?

Medical experts estimate that anywhere from four percent to 20 percent of the general population has MVP, with women more affected than men. It also tends to run in families. Why does MVP appear in this book as a differential diagnosis with CFIDS? The incidence of MVP is significant-ly higher in CFIDS patients. It may be that the ubiquitous yeast cell has something to do with this. The liver is the first organ invaded by the yeast cell. The yeast cell can use the extensive venous connection between liver and heart to spread itself to the mitral valve and contribute to its leaking. Your doctor might think that MVP is the *cause* of your fatigue and not take further measures to look for other causes. With the information in this book, you don't have to stop at a diagnosis of MVP. You can continue to look for other possible elements involved in your CFIDS.

* What to Do About MVP

First, a cardiologist (referred by your family doctor or internist) should determine the extent of the mitral valve leak by doing an echocardiogram. If the valve defect is minor, it becomes debatable whether your doctor will prescribe antibiotics when you undergo a medical or dental procedure. Most dentists will not perform any procedure on MVP patients unless they take preventive antibiotics (given before and after the procedure).

While the danger of infective endocarditis with patients who have a serious leaky valve is very real, CFIDS patients whose other symptoms will be aggravated by antibiotics face a dilemma. It is a judgment call to be made in tandem by the dentist and patient. If you take antibiotics, then be sure to take acidophilus products to protect your intestinal flora and double your intake of antifungal therapy when you are suffering from yeast overgrowth. (See Chapters Six and Nine for more information on yeast infections and their treatments.)

If you have been diagnosed with MVP, you should be periodically reexamined to see whether the condition has worsened. There is usually no prohibition against exercise for the majority óf MVP patients.

Besides the specific tests for CFIDS and ruling out the possibility of other, more serious disorders, you may need tests for underlying viral, yeast or parasitic conditions. As the following four chapters describe, any of these conditions are consequences of a suppressed immune system.

Your doctor will need to rule out viral, yeast and parasitic involvement before your treatment can begin. Once the reasons for your illness are pinpointed, the next section looks at treatments.

References:
1. "Chronic Fatigue Syndrome and the Diagnostic Utility of Antibody to Epstein-Barr Virus Early Antigen," Walter Hellinger, M.D., et al., Mayo Clinic, *Journal of the American Medical Association*, Vol. 260, No. 7, pages 971-973.
2. "Hypersensitivity to Vaginal Candidiasis or Treatment Vehicles in the Pathogenesis of Minor Vestibular Gland Syndrome." Stanley Marinoff, MD, Maria Turner MD; From the Dept. of Obstetrics and Gynecology and of Dermatology, George Washington University, Washington D.C., *Journal of Reproductive Medicine*, Vol. 31, No. 9, September 1986.
3. "Therapeutic Studies on Vulvar Vestibulitis"; by Eduard Friedrich, Jr., M.D., from the Dept. of Obstetrics and Gynecology, University of Florida College of Medicine, Gainesville; *The Journal of Reproductive Medicine*, Vol. 33, No. 6, June, 1988.

CHAPTER FIVE

VIRUSES: EVER-PRESENT AND ALL-POWERFUL

Marc, 34 years old, looked puzzled and pale as he entered the doctor's office. He had been under tremendous stress with a very demanding and unrewarding job. When his fiancé broke up with him, he came down with the flu. But three weeks later, he still felt achy, with a sore throat and swollen lymph nodes. To compound his misery, for the first time in years, he had a recurrent attack of sexual herpes. Despite high doses of Zovirax ™, the indicated medication for his genital herpes, Marc experienced only limited relief. He felt more fatigued as time went on. His family doctor prescribed some antibiotics which at first seemed to help, but his persistent sore throat did not respond to further administration of various antibiotics.

Marc felt depressed and so exhausted that he needed a nap every afternoon. When Epstein-Barr and Cytomegalovirus blood levels were obtained, they showed some acute reactivation. Once this became clear, Marc was put on a program of rest, proper nutrition and supplements which turned the tide for his physical symptoms. He began consulting a psychotherapist and was able to drastically change his lifestyle to one with less pressure. Marc has been able to stay symptom-free after that last viral bout.

"It's a virus." How many times have you heard those words from your doctor? You go into the office feeling ill, perhaps with fever, intestinal discomfort and muscle weakness. And your doctor usually says, "there's nothing I can give you to make it go away. Take these medicines to ease your symptoms."

Viruses are responsible for many illnesses: the "common" cold (there are more than 200 varieties of cold viruses!), influenza, or flu, chicken pox, measles, warts, shingles, intestinal disorders and Mononucleosis.

Forgetting momentarily the suffering they cause, viruses are magnificent little structures. When the electronic microscope was invented in 1931, researchers got their chance to look at the myriad shapes — spherical, lunar, football and soccer ball shapes — formed by these organisms. All viruses have the same basic structure: a core of genetic material (either a DNA or RNA molecule) surrounded by a protective protein shell. (See Figure 6). Unlike other creatures, the virus cannot metabolize nutrients — it cannot feed itself. It depends entirely on the help of the host cell. Once activated, the viral genes reorder the host cell to begin producing more viruses. These new viruses will be carbon copies of the original invader. Scientists have harnessed this mechanism to create vaccines and substances by putting the virus to work to replicate itself. Although the virus, when attached to the host cell, is a veritable production line, it cannot multiply itself alone.

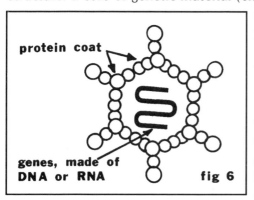

Typical structure of a virus, showing the core, or nucleus, comprised of genetic material, and the outer protein coat

So the virus needs the help of your body to do its work. Without the cooperation of the weakened defense system, the virus becomes powerless. Although acute viral infections like influenza kill thousands of people each year — especially the elderly and children — most people are able to defeat these tiny invaders. Fever, chills, swollen lymph glands and itchy rashes are due to the vigorous activity of the immune system, in a merciless battle with these viruses.

Other viruses have a different approach. Between attacks, they will lie dormant in the body, waiting like vultures to reactivate in moments when the host's immune system is suppressed. Herpes simplex viruses are a good example of this tactic. The hiding places are different; the herpes zoster virus, which causes chicken pox, sometimes hides in nerve cells and can cause — years after the initial pox attack — the excruciating pain of shingles. The Epstein-Barr virus, or herpes Simplex III, hides in the B-cells, the very cells that make antibodies to viruses. It is the Trojan horse in the body!

Medical researchers are currently trying to make vaccinations from restructured viruses, thereby creating remedies, so desperately needed in the battle against viral diseases. Some vaccinations have been extremely successful, such as the polio, measles and rubella vaccines. But viruses have the ability to change in structure, constantly creating mutations that can escape the killing effect of vaccines. This is especially the case with the ever-changing character of the influenza ("flu") epidemics.

In this chapter, I will briefly describe the common viral illnesses associated with CFIDS, their symptoms and their proper diagnoses.

Epstein-Barr and CMV - The Tricky Viruses

Epstein-Barr virus and Cytomegalovirus (CMV) are present in 80% of the population. Both EBV and CMV are members of the herpes family of viruses, which cause chicken pox, cold sores, genital lesions, shingles, and other ailments. All these viruses are tricky. They have the habit of hiding out in the body in a latent, or inactive state. Then they get reactivated and attack, typically when the body's resistance is low. That's what happened in Marc's case. But even in this elusive company, the Epstein-Barr virus stands out as the most eccentric and fascinating herpes of them all.

Investigations have shown that EBV is widely disseminated throughout the world. Blood samples collected from isolated tribes in the Amazon rain forests have proved free of measles antibodies but tested positive for Epstein-Barr. The virus is easily passed along in the saliva, which explains its ubiquity. Oddly enough, the consequences of contracting the virus vary dramatically from place to place and culture to culture. In the United States and Europe, it causes the "kissing disease," or mononucleosis. In Africa, it is involved with Burkitt's Lymphoma, a fast-growing tumor of the jaw, which often leads to death. EBV seems to be also closely implicated with cancers like Kaposi's sarcoma and multiple sclerosis. In Asia, the same virus has been linked to nasopharyngeal (nose and throat) cancer.

Co-Factors Determine How Sick You Get

Why does the same virus lead to all these different clinical results? Part of the answer lies in what we call "co-factors." Burkitt's Lymphoma, for example, appears in a belt across central Africa marked by high rainfall and warm temperatures — the precise features of mosquito country. The co-factor allowing the virus to trigger Burkitt's Lymphoma seems to be a weakening of the immune system brought on by constant exposure to malaria and yellow fever. And, according to the Chinese, **humidity** is **the** climatic factor that most weakens the immune system.

In the case of mononucleosis, the key co-factor is age. In general, a toddler exposed to the Epstein-Barr virus will develop antibodies and never exhibit so much as a sniffle. An older child may have a mild sore throat for a day or two. But a young adult encountering the virus for the first time stands a better than even chance of spending a truly miserable month in bed with mono. Obviously, if early exposure to the virus confers a kind of immunity, conventional ideas about hygiene don't hold up. In Indonesia and Mexico, where nearly all children have EBV in their bloodstream by age six, infectious mononucleosis is unheard of. But in Sweden or England, where parents are fastidious about kissing, many infants and young children don't get exposed; as a result they develop mono as teenagers.

Suppressed Immune System - The Common Denominator

Because EBV is so omnipresent, the Centers for Disease Control (CDC) and many doctors are leery of reports of widespread new epidemics of CFIDS, with involvement of viruses such as EBV. After all, how can you have an epidemic of a disease when everybody already has antibodies in their bloodstream?

One reason is the common denominator of a suppressed immune system, as a result of the triggering factors discussed in Chapter Two. Another co-factor is the simultaneous presence of the other herpes simplex viruses, such as h. simplex I (cold sores), h. simplex II (genital herpes) and h. simplex IV, or CMV. Now if you have the latent presence of these viruses in your body, with occasional flare-ups, this causes continuous onslaughts against the strength of your immune system.

When your immune system becomes exhausted, retroviruses can creep up on you without warning. Like other viruses, retroviruses cannot replicate without taking over and exploiting a cell. What is unique about retroviruses is their capacity to reverse the ordinary flow of genetic information stored in the cell's nucleus, or center. The genetic material of a retrovirus is RNA. The retrovirus carries an enzyme to use the viral RNA for making DNA.

Perhaps the least understood and least accepted co-factor is the presence of candida albicans, a common yeast cell. This microorganism is extensively discussed in the next chapter. In common practice I have seen that even for patients with confirmed CFIDS, candida was present well before reactivation of Herpes Simplex viruses.

How EBV Works: Its Tricks

The primary EBV infection occurs orally. The virus infects the B lymphocytes of the immune system, our white blood cells formed in the bone marrow that normally manufacture antibodies vigorously.

Then the immune system responds by producing a legion of activated killer T-cells. During the course of the infection, you may feel horribly sick, since your immune system is literally at war with itself. This is the "Herxheimer reaction," which is the cleansing phase of the battle. During this cleansing, toxins are released. You experience this process with the appearance of flu-like symptoms: headaches, muscle and joint pains, and fatigue for one to two days after your body starts killing off bacteria, viruses or yeast cells.

It sounds paradoxical, but the process of getting well at the microbial level temporarily makes you feel sicker than ever. So, the Herxheimer reaction is actually a sign that you are getting better. This is important to keep in mind as you begin to experience the symptoms of CFIDS. You often feel worse before you feel better. And it's a good idea not to think in terms of a "quick fix." There is no magic pill to make you feel better instantly.

Once you get well, the threat of EBV reactivation doesn't disappear. A few transformed B-cells harboring the virus — about one in a million— remain present in otherwise healthy individuals. It is like a slow, incessant battle between T-cells and a few virus-infected B-cells, neither party claiming victory. And with virtually all previously infected healthy individuals thus far analyzed, a surprisingly high frequency of specific memory cells can be found in their blood. This really means that there is a continuous war-truce going on, a state of high alert, easily erupting into a full-fledged battle when the co-factors discussed above intervene.

The Symptoms of Viral Disease

It isn't easy to confirm diagnosis of a viral disease. That's because the symptoms have such variety and at the same time are nonspecific. Who hasn't suffered from fatigue, some depression or muscle pain? To make matters worse, another condition, candidiasis, shares many of the same symptoms. But to really confound the doctor, both EBV and candidiasis can exist simultaneously in 75% of the cases as epiphenomena of CFIDS. Of course, there are laboratory tests to help distinguish between the two conditions. Even so, lab tests aren't the deciding factor. Clinically, however, it is possible to distinguish between candidiasis and viral disease, if both don't exist together. This will be shown in Chapter Six, on candida.

Key Symptoms

The following key symptoms and characteristics should be present at sometime during the course of the illness:
* *Muscle pain or weakness upon exercising.* This is different from the normal muscle fatigue experienced after exercise. This fatigue will inhibit the patient from exercising.
* Symptoms may appear intermittently; you may often experience a relapse.
* Exhaustion.
* Unusual muscle fatigue: this is often referred to in medicine as fibromyositis (inflammation of the muscle fiber), and is characterized by muscle spasm, painful knots and muscles that feel like lead, especially in the neck area.
* A history of the symptoms lasting more than three months. In addition to these key symptoms, there is a group of common symptoms, which can, but do not have to, exist at some time during the course of the disease. Often patients and doctors mistakenly conclude that if the patients have not had sore throats, they can't possibly have viral disease.

Common Symptoms

* "Brain fog":
This is an inability to concentrate and remember simple things. For instance, some people with this symptom have to read a passage three times before it makes sense to them. Patients forget the names of their close friends, or can't balance their checkbooks.

This "brain fog" fluctuates in character and intensity. Patients never know when it is going to hit them, which creates much anxiety, especially when it occurs in professional people with high degrees of responsibility. This symptom can also express itself in a lack of coordination, excessive drowsiness and balance disturbance. If you did not know better, you might diagnose these as victims of Alzheimer's disease.

* Muscle symptoms:

This is the most important symptom in identifying viral involvement with CFIDS. In the case of people with EBV, CMV or HHV-6, even short periods of exercise cause muscle fatigue and exhaustion. The patient needs to recuperate for a full day or more! This is not the case when parasites or yeast reactivation are present. For these people, exercise makes them feel better and they are able to resume their exercise programs the next day.

Intermittent muscle twitching and delayed muscle recovery are also common symptoms of viral disease. Muscle twitching of the eyes is very disturbing to the patient and can become visible to other people. Twitching of bigger muscle groups in arms or legs, called fasciculations, is often present and easily recognized.

* Infectious Symptoms:

These include recurrent sore throats, recurrent colds and painful, swollen lymph glands in the neck.

* Psychological symptoms:

Patients often experience depression and severe mood swings — one can feel fine at 10 a.m., yet be totally depressed at 2 p.m. Anger and irritability are also common symptoms. Of course, the lack of support from family and doctors only adds fuel to the fire, completing the vicious circle: the patient is more likely to become increasingly angry and despairing.

* Gastrointestinal symptoms:

These symptoms are usually minimal with viral involvement. Symptoms such as irritable bowel syndrome, excessive gas and bloating, as well as constipation, are more likely linked to a generalized yeast infection. See the next chapter for a discussion of this.

Making the Diagnosis

To make the diagnosis of viral involvement, the doctor should first and foremost be noting your symptoms and your appearance. However, diagnosis can become complicated clinically because so many of the symptoms of viral illness are also common with other immune-suppressed diseases, such as candidiasis, parasitical disease, or AIDS. Remember, all these diseases have a common origin: the suppressed immune system. Only the intensity of the symptoms differs.

There are available laboratory tests which your doctor may use to help in his or her diagnosis. This being the case, it is somewhat helpful to be able to fall back on laboratory tests that are available. In this section of the chapter, you will become acquainted with several of these viral tests. Keep in mind that they are still not very sensitive in picking up viruses, but if you have some knowledge of what they were designed for, perhaps you can become a more helpful partner in your own health care.

EBV Antibody Titers

EBV antibody titers (levels) are tests indicating the body's response to EBV antigens, which are complex substances produced by the virus during different stages of replication. Antigens serve as markers for your body's defense system. The immune system recognizes antigens as being foreign. Once EBV enters the body, its antigens stimulate the production of antibodies — proteins carried in the blood to respond to infection.

By measuring the levels of antibodies in your blood, the tests will show to what extent you have been exposed to the virus, and what stage that exposure is at currently. For instance, depending on the antibody level detected, the lab test will show whether your illness had a recent onset, or whether you are on the way to recovery.

EBV antibody levels are obtained from about 5 cc of blood taken from your vein. Although laboratories performing these tests present the results in slightly different ways, the levels of antigens found in your blood are recorded in four parts:

* VCA-IgG
* IgM, or Anti-Viral Capsid Antigen
* EAD, or Anti-Early Antigen Diffuse Component
* EBNA, or Epstein-Barr Anti-Nuclear Antigen

The interpretation of EBV antibody levels is based on the following premises:

1. Once a person becomes infected with EBV, the anti-VCA antibodies appear first.

2. Anti-EA antibodies appear next, or are present with anti-VCA antibodies early in the course of illness. Active disease is

indicated when the anti-EA levels are higher than those in people who have recovered from infection and have no symptoms.

3. As the patient recovers, anti-VCA and anti-EA antibodies decrease, and anti-EBNA antibodies appear. Anti-EBNA reflects a past infection.

4. After the patient is well, anti-VCA and anti-EBNA are always present. These levels persist for life, but usually in lower ranges than those appearing in acute illness.

The above findings are reflected in Table 2 below. The "reference rate" refers to the normal rate of appearance of the corresponding antibody in the left-hand column. For instance, the normal level of IgG anti-Viral Capsid AG is less than 1/100. In the patient's results, the number is 270, indicating infection with EBV. The interpretation of the blood test comprises the second part of this table.

TABLE #2

EXAMPLE OF EPSTEIN-BARR VIRUS ANTIBODY

PANELOF ITL ELISA VALUES

MEASUREMENT	REFERENCE RATE	PATIENTS RESULTS
IgG-Anti-Viral Capsid Ag	Less than 1/100	270
IgM-Anti-Viral Capsid Ag	Less than 1/50	30
IgG-Anti-Early Antigen	Less than 1/20	25
IgG-Anti-Nuclear Ag	Less than 1/100	130
IgM-Anti-Nuclear Ag	Less than 1/50	60

What does your doctor look for?

INTERPRETATIONS OF SEROLOGY PATTERNS
IN EBV INFECTION
Patient's EBV Status

Antibodies	Primary	EBV	Convalescent(3 mo.)	Past	Reactivated
VCA-IgM	+	+ or -	+ or -	-	-
VCA-IgG	+	+	+	+	+
EA-IgG	-	+	+	-	+
EBNA-IgG	-	+ or -	+ or -	+	+
EBNA-IgM	+	+ or -	+ or -	-	+

In the above example, the patient has a reactivation of the virus.

The above explanation should help doctors determine whether their patients have a past or present infection. The EBV antibody test is complex and undoubtedly, will be replaced in the future by even more sensitive tests. So far, the test performed by Immuno Tech Laboratories is the most sensitive one.

Other worthwhile tests to be done are antibody titers against CMV (the same interpretation as for EBV), Coxsackie B viruses, HHV-6, and Herpes simplex I and II, since they reactivate often at the same time as EBV in CFIDS patients. These tests are worthwhile because these viruses often group together to attack your immune system. Determination of their levels will show to what extent your immune system is under siege.

The probability of yet another kind of virus playing a role in the origin of CFIDS was investigated by immunologist Eileen De Freitas, in conjunction with doctors David Bell and Paul Cheney. On September 4, 1990, they presented a paper to the 11th International Congress of Neuropathology in Kyoto, Japan, entitled "Evidence of Retrovirus in Patients with CFIDS." In approximately 75% of CFIDS sufferers studied by De Freitas and her colleagues, there was evidence of a retrovirus, resembling HTLV-2, the AIDS virus, but slightly different from the prototype discovered by Dr. Robert Gallo, a co-discoverer of the AIDS virus, several years ago. Whereas EBV and HHV-6, or Human Herpes Virus-6, another of the herpes family, are felt to be ubiquitous, this retrovirus is present in very minute proportions in the population. However, De Freitas, et al. were very careful not to implicate this new retrovirus as the cause of CFIDS. Patients with suppressed immune systems have reactivation of herpes viruses (EBV, CMV, HHV-6, Herpes Zoster), and these viruses are consequences, not causes of CFIDS, as figure 1 in Chapter Two showed.

Could it be that this retrovirus, isolated from CFIDS patients, is another epiphenomena? It could well be. And the fact that this retrovirus is less prevalent in the general population (especially in comparison with the herpes viruses) may indicate that the immune system has to be compromised before the retrovirus can penetrate the defense mechanisms. Or is this virus weakening the immune systems first and therefore allowing herpes viruses to reactivate? A careful study of these patients' histories, in which triggering factors discussed in Chapter Two are taken into account, might answer this question. Only then will scientists know the difference between causation and consequence. In the meantime, finding another virus does not give much hope to present sufferers. Fabrication of a vaccination, according to the researchers, could take up to six years, and that could only help people who are not infected at the moment. Is finding this retrovirus a research breakthrough? If we can show causality, yes. If not, then it is just another "EBV or CMV."

This chapter has described viruses and the symptoms and diagnostic testing for viral disease. For treatment of these illnesses, turn to Chapter Nine. The next chapter will discuss a condition which may be responsible for more than you give it credit for — yeast infections.

Footnote:

Very sensitive tests are performed by Immunotech Laboratories (ITL). Their diagnostic test panels for CFIDS include EB virus antibody, candida antibody profile, T and B cells, Herpes 1 and 2, CMV antibody and human herpes virus 6 antibody.

ITL
1185 Linda Vista Drive
San Marcos, CA 92069
1-800-848-2546, or (619) 744-7340.

CHAPTER SIX

CANDIDA GROWS BY LEAPS AND BOUNDS

Myriam, a 27-year-old high school science teacher, was plagued with relentless fatigue. To her consternation, she had a hard time remembering simple things such as her friends' names. Puzzled by this almost overnight change, she realized when she consulted her physician that this condition had started when she began to take birth control pills and entered a new relationship. She later suffered from vaginal yeast infections or urinary tract infections the day after sexual intercourse.

Her premenstrual symptoms had always included painful, swollen breasts, but now she also experienced increased mood swings and uncontrollable cravings for sweets. The doctors she consulted prescribed either vaginal creams or suppositories and antibiotics for the alleged urinary infections. However, all her symptoms intensified and by the time she consulted our office, she was depressed and frustrated. A candida antibody test showed a high amount of IgM antibodies, indicating a recent yeast infection.

After a few weeks on a yeast-free diet, an antifungal medication and intake of acidophilus, together with stopping the pill, Myriam's symptoms cleared up completely. Myriam found another method of contraception (Footnote #1) and continues to follow an improved, sugar free diet. In her case, the triggering factor for her yeast infection was taking birth control pills, together with increased sexual activity.

It is hard to believe that these tiny microflora or yeast cells can play such havoc with our bodies. Normally yeast cells live in harmony with other bacteria in a concentration composed of millions of bacteria versus perhaps one candida cell. These bacteria form the normal flora of the gastrointestinal tract and inhibit the overgrowth of yeast in normal circumstances. We will see in the next pages what triggering factors turn these innocent-looking creatures into vultures, what symptoms they cause with overgrowth and how we can detect them. Finally, in Chapter Nine, you'll see what your most successful battle plan will be.

Candida albicans is a yeast-like fungus that is found in the mucous membranes of warm-blooded animals and humans. In individuals whose immune systems are intact, the organism is typically benign, but fueled by the triggering factors discussed in Chapter Two, candida albicans tends to overgrow in the body. If left unchecked, it can cause a very serious condition, systemic candidiasis, causing an array of symptoms and leading to other immuno-suppressed conditions when not corrected.

Candida albicans is present right now in people's systems in much higher amounts than we thought. In fact, the increasing growth of yeast cells is the most important consequence or epiphenomena of a debililated immune system. The yeast cell is a lot more opportunistic than most of the viruses. The overgrowth of yeast is a consequence of dramatic changes that have occurred in our environment, our food intake and our emotional lives. All these triggering factors have caused depleted immune systems, a virtual open invitation to overgrowth of candida albicans.

Some physicians discount candidiasis as a true condition, comparing it to other "fad" diagnoses, such as hypoglycemia which was prevalent in the 70's. Facing a complicated set of symptoms, most doctors may ask for a routine blood panel, which, with the exception of slight anemia and a decreased amount of white blood cells, turns out to be normal. More sophisticated tests must be conducted to pick up yeast overgrowth. When a doctor does not consider the possibility of candidiasis it is unlikely that he or she will even ask for such a test. So the patient is told "on paper you look perfectly healthy," and, it is implied, there is no reason for you to feel sick.

This chapter is designed to help you find out whether your symptoms match those seen in candidiasis patients, and help you find the right diagnostic tests. Then, in Chapter Nine, you'll find the recommended therapies to treat this condition.

Do These Symptoms Sound Familiar?

Diagnosis of yeast overgrowth is not easy. There is a broad pattern of symptoms which are often not linked because the patient sees a specialist for each set of symptoms. For instance, Gloria consults her gynecologist for a vaginal yeast infection. She is prescribed an antifungal cream or vaginal tablets to take. The vaginal discharge seems to disappear after 5-6 days but recurs with her next menstrual cycle or right after sexual intercourse, as in Myriam's case.

Then things get out of hand: after numerous further episodes of vaginal discharge, Gloria is still not free from this curse. The doctor may not be able to find any cause for her condition. But perhaps she had had some minor surgery just before the first attack. The surgery was complicated by an infection and logically, broad-spectrum antibiotics, given intravenously, were administered for five days. Adding to these events might be additional stress at work and at home. Often, the gynecologist will not link all these events with the patient's yeast infections. Gloria will probably get tired of using all those vaginal creams. So, she may be referred to yet another specialist.

Consider an alternative scenario: Alice suddenly finds she had multiple food allergies, which cause bloating, excess gas and stomach distension. She may have alternating attacks of constipation and diarrhea. Her physician starts with an x-ray of the bowels, which shows a "spastic colon," a kind of catch-all phrase for a symptomatic condition. Medication does not help, and now, Alice becomes really concerned: she is gaining weight, she is constantly hungry and she has incredible cravings for sugar and other carbohydrates. Getting out of bed in the morning seems to be an impossible task, and if it were not for her cup of coffee, she would never make it to work. Depression and mood swings are the next step. Her family gets fed up with her "asocial" behavior and her chronic fatigue, which they label "laziness."

These two women most probably suffer from candidiasis. Another group of people prone to yeast overgrowth are alcoholics. Because of the sugar content in alcohol, yeast cells multiply quickly in their bodies. Even when they are in recovery, the yeast overgrowth continues, as the alcohol addiction is replaced by an addiction to sugar and coffee. The psychological support recovering alcoholics get from their peers will not suppress the growth of the yeast cells, creating incredible cravings for carbohydrates. There is a physical dependency, which has to be corrected by a yeast-free diet, acidophilus and yeast-killing drugs. Some recovering alcoholics have simply replaced one addiction — alcohol — with another: sugar.

Other Symptoms

Even though the following paragraphs talk about symptoms common to most candidiasis sufferers, you should not compare yourself to others with this condition. If you gathered a hundred people with the condition, you would have one hundred distinct cases and gradations of symptoms. This is due in part to the fact that people are subjected to different triggering factors — hereditary, emotional, nutritional and environmental.

Those suffering from yeast overgrowth will often experience an irritation and burning feeling of all the mucous membranes — around the anus, the vagina, the mouth and the lips, and even the lining of the stomach, which creates a constant feeling of hunger. These symptoms are often accompanied by attacks of cystitis, which is an inflammation of the urinary bladder with frequent, urgent and burning urination. These urinary infections are most commonly treated with antibiotics, although often urine cultures come back clear. However, the "infections" seem to recur with regularity. And they are accompanied by symptoms of "brain fog," which limits the patient's concentration and short-term memory.

Anxiety attacks are an especially frightening experience, and can occur even though the patient is in therapy. While some physicians may look for psychological triggering factors, these anxiety attacks can be caused by the accumulation of toxins, released by die-off. As described earlier, "die-off" is the release of toxins caused by the battle between white blood cells and the microorganism (virus, bacteria, yeast, parasite) which is present. So, the die-off phenomenon is the clean-up of the battlefield.

These anxiety attacks can be intensified at night. When we sleep, we don't have bowel movements or urinate, we don't sweat or move much. So our bodies have none of the usual ways to get rid of toxins. Usually, using an enema or taking high doses of Vitamin C powder (1 tsp every hour) will clear these attacks.

Many candidiasis symptoms are caused by the build-up of toxins in the body. Another common symptom is the metallic taste patients experience. It often accompanies severe constipation and dry, itchy skin, which are symptoms of toxicity and heat in the body. When those patients drink water, even it has a metallic taste. This unpleasant symptom disappears when there is a good evacuation of the toxins.

Most people suffering from yeast overgrowth will show several of the above symptoms at some point in the course of their disease. You may have the impression that only women suffer from yeast overgrowth. This is not true. Men can also show most of the above symptoms. Prostatitis (inflammation of the prostate), the homologue of vaginitis, often is a first and unsuspected symptom. Of course, any man with prostatitis should be examined by a doctor and the possibility of malignancy ruled out.

You may be noticing some common threads here. Symptoms experienced by candidiasis patients are similar to those of viral diseases, discussed in the last chapter. Even ARC and AIDS patients have some of these same conditions.

Remembering Figure 1 on page 27, CFIDS is the umbrella for all these conditions, so CFIDS patients have most of the symptoms described in this chapter. Keep in mind that the root of all these conditions is a suppressed immune system. The symptoms are those of a weak immune system, although they vary in degree.

However, it is possible to clinically distinguish the symptoms of candidiasis from those of viral diseases. Table 3 compares the two diseases by symptom to show you whether they differ.

Common Candidiasis and Viral Symptoms

There are no rules to determine how many of these symptoms have to be present to warrant a diagnosis of candidiasis, viral illness or even CFIDS. You have to be vigilant in noticing the changes in your health. The perceived symptoms, combined with the known triggering factors, will give you enough evidence for consulting your doctor.

1. "Brain fog": definite symptom in both conditions; difficulty concentrating, short-term memory disturbances; similar to an early stage of Alzheimer's.
2. Irritability, drowsiness, blurred vision, skin pallor, or cold extremities and extreme fatigue are all common symptoms.
3. Insomnia, headaches, mood swings and depression.
4. Sensation of head swelling.
5. Weak, shaky muscles
6. Frequent sore throats
7. Unexplained crying spells
8. Irritability
9. Chest congestion and palpitations

10. Feeling of being crazy or falling apart
11. Shortness of breath
12. Chills and low-grade fevers
14. Hypersensitivity towards sunlight, sound and touch

The following is a list of symptoms and their presence or absence in viral diseases or candidiasis.

TABLE 3

COMPARISON OF SYMPTOMS IN
VIRAL DISEASES AND CANDIDIASIS

VIRAL DISEASES	CANDIDIASIS
1. Intermittent attacks, at least in beginning of the disease	1. Progressive, worsening condition
2. No cravings for carbohydrates	2. Irresistible sugar cravings
3. Few gastrointestinal signs	3. Constipation, gas, bloating, stomach pain
4. No food sensitivities	4. Extreme food sensitivities
5. No skin rashes or nail infections	5. Butterfly rash on face, nail infections
6. No postnasal drip	6. Constant postnasal drip
7. No hormonal influence	7. Premenstrual worsening amenorrhea, menstrual irregularities
8. Symptoms worse with exercise	8. Symptoms better with exercise

VIRAL DISEASES	CANDIDIASIS
9. No environmental sensitivities	9. Environmental sensitivities, 60% of the time
10. No cystitis attacks	10. Recurrent cystitis
11. No aggravation of symptoms in damp weather	11. Aggravation on damp, foggy days
12. No itching	12. Itching all over the body, esp. anal/vaginal itching
13. Changes on tongue (redness, cracks) are on the tip	13. Yellow, white fur in middle of tongue
14. No vaginal or urethral discharge	14. Discharge present
15. No thrush seen	15. Thrush, can be present
16. No anemia/hypothyroidea	16. Frequent anemia, hypothyroidea
17. Chiropractic adjustments hold	17. Patient cannot hold adjustment; patient is out of alignment one hour after adjustment.

Keep in mind that viral diseases and candidiasis can go together in about 75% of cases, creating a full-blown picture of CFIDS. These "mixed" infections make it difficult for the doctor to distinguish one condition from another. However, an experienced clinician will be able to make the distinction. And, of course, there are always the laboratory tests.

Accurately Diagnosing Candidiasis

In diagnosing candidiasis, your clinical picture, or set of symptoms, is the most important. You filled in the questionnaire in

Chapter One. That mentioned information about triggering factors and symptoms which will provide your doctor with important details about your condition. Take this questionnaire with you when you visit your doctor.

The Laboratory Tests

* Increased frequency of yeast cells, isolated from sputum, urine, or feces cultures, should lead a physician to suspect candidiasis in high-risk individuals. It is important to know that these tests will almost never be sensitive enough to come out positive.

* A purged stool test (Dowell Laboratories, Mesa, AZ), can show the presence of yeast, but only when the yeast is abundant. However, a negative purged stool test does not exclude presence of yeast in the blood.

* Improvements in blood culture methods promise diagnostic gains. This is potentially the most useful yeast isolation, but it is frequently unrewarding. In patients with invasive candidiasis, up to 25% lack detectable antibodies to candida. In other words, these people will have a *negative* blood test in spite of the presence of the disease.

The Candida Antibody Blood Test

The principle of this test is that candida albicans, in normal circumstances, is present only in the gastrointestinal tract. The moment candida cells arrive in the bloodstream, they are recognized (by the lymphocytes) as strange objects; hence, antibodies are formed.

In the candida antibody test, three kinds of antibodies are measured: IgM, IgA and IgG. The IgM antibody is the first antibody to form, peaking two weeks after exposure to the yeast cells, then quickly disappearing. The IgG appears by the third day and will be the highest figure you get. However, if a person is chronically exposed, which is the case with most candidiasis patients, IgG AND IgA will give a response; there will be no IgM.

Considerable effort has been devoted to the serodiagnosis of candida albicans over the last ten years. Generally, confirmation for diagnosis of systemic candidiasis has been based on culturing the organisms. However, false negative cultures are common, and the ubiquitous nature of candida in the human flora frequently results in the isolation of the organism from peripheral blood, and does not necessarily imply a diagnosis of invasive candidiasis. A number of serolgic tests have been used for the detection of candida infections, but reports are conflicting on the diagnostic value of such tests. The confusion about serodiagnosis results from differences in specificity and sensitivity. Many of the available tests will show significant candida antibody titers among healthy individuals. Worse yet, some of the available tests consistently are negative even when patients have serious candida infections. You can imagine the confusion among practitioners in choosing a valid blood test. And for a lot of patients, whether they will be treated for yeast overgrowth or not, will depend on a positive blood test.

Fischer and colleagues (1985-Ref.1) have shown that the more sensitive ELISA method employing the cytoplasmatic antigen, has a sensitivity and specificity of *greater than* 90%. In addition, measurement of class specific antibodies (anti-candida IgG, IgA, and IgM) may have diagnostic value (Schonheyder et al., 1983, 1987-Ref.2). Immuno Tech Laboratories (7800 S. Elati, Littleton, CO 80120. Tel. (303) 798-4751 and (800) 628-5008) presently has the most reliable serological test available for diagnosing candida infections. The very sensitive ELISA method is used to quantitate serum levels of IgG, IgA, and IgM specific for candida cytoplasmatic antigen. Elevated IgM levels are generally indicative of an early inapparent infection. Increased IgG levels are associated with acute or chronic infections, especially when accompanied by elevated IgA levels. Successful treatment usually results in a fairly rapid decrease in specific IgA antibody levels. As you can see, patients owe it to themselves to ask for this specific test, performed by Immuno Tech Laboratories, in order to avoid false negative diagnosis and needless expense.

You might ask, knowing what you know about antibody formation and immunity, "Why don't those antibodies that appear in viral diseases and candidiasis protect us from further infection?" The answer is because these antibodies do not kill. The killing is done by "natural killer cells" (NK cells), while antibodies are a reflection of the activity of our immune system.

How Did Candida A. Get This Far?

All the triggers — hereditary factors, nutritional factors, emotional and environmental factors — leading to a depressed immune system can be responsible for an overgrowth of yeast cells (See Chapter Two). However, there are some factors which really stand out as responsible for the overgrowth of candida albicans.

External Factors

When our first antibiotics, namely, penicillin, became available during WWII, medicine had indisputably taken a big step forward. But things got somewhat out of hand after that initial period. Broad-spectrum antibiotics were l/m and are — used for common colds so that the normal flora of the intestine (coli, bacteroides and enterobacteria) can be suppressed. We all know of the use of tetracyclines in the therapy of acne; low doses were, and still are, given for months at a time. In a few days, this results in a replacement of the normal flora with one that consists of resistant organisms, including the yeast.

Ampicillin and bactrim are frequently given because patients insist on strong medication for a cold, since they have no time (due to life's constraints) to heal more naturally. The "time-is-money" attitude which dictates this behavior is not necessarily the wisest long term approach, as we are discovering.

"I never took antibiotics in my life," you may say. Most likely you have, but didn't know it. Adding low doses of antibiotics to the feed of chickens, cows and pigs is routinely done. People who raise cows or pigs insist that they must use antibiotics to prevent infections and promote growth of the animals. However, the regular feeding of antibiotics to livestock may produce resistant bacteria and lead to their multiplication in the flesh of animals. This resistance to antibiotics is transferable to the person ingesting the meat of these animals.

Antibiotics are not the only "magic bullets" leading to yeast infections. Other factors are also well-recognized as creating opportunities for the conversion of candida species from an innocent existence into a pathogen, invading all the tissues and organs. Cortisone preparations cause a fluctuation in the peripheral lymphocytes, exerting an immuno-suppressive effect that increases the risk of candidiasis. Cytotoxic drugs used in cancer therapy cause a decrease in the white blood cells and will suppress the bone marrow, which is the production center of the body's defenders. The management of these patients allows organisms like candida to invade the deep tissues.

Birth control pills, in use since 1952, create other opportunities for candida. "The Pill" alters the vaginal secretions, elevating the glycogen (sugar) content, which favors the growth of candida. And other forms of birth control can be just as harmful. (For more on this, see Footnote 1 at the end of the chapter.)

Hormonal fluctuations in the third trimester of pregnancy also alter the vaginal secretions, elevating the glycogen content which again favors the growth of candida. Since this is a frequent condition of pregnancy, this yeast overgrowth can be passed to the baby. The progesterone increase before the menstrual cycle will increase the sugar content in the blood, again enhancing the multiplication of yeast cells. No wonder women get irresistible food cravings. Their bodies are prone to overgrowth of yeast cells, which sets up these uncontrollable urges.

As if this is not enough, other medical conditions favor the growth of candida: burns, surgical interventions, indwelling catheters, hypothyroidism, ferriprive anemia and adult diabetes mellitus; conditions that have to be corrected in order to conquer the yeast completely.

You can visualize how yeast cells proliferate in the body by turning to "Autobiography of a Yeast Cell," which appears in the Appendix at the back of the book. And in Chapter Nine, you'll read about therapy for yeast overgrowth, which can make as big a difference in your life as it did in Myriam's.

In the next chapter, you will learn about parasites, the "forgotten" diagnosis!

REFERENCES
(1). "Disseminated Candidiasis; A comparison of two immunologic techniques in the diagnosis." by Fischer et al., *American Towers of Medical Sciences* 290: 135-141 (1985)
(2). "IgA and IgG serum antibodies to candida albicans in women of child-bearing Age." by Schonheider et al., *Sabouradia* 21:223-231 (1983)

Footnote:
1. Spermicidal creams and foams, used with or without a diaphragm, increase the risk of recurrent yeast and cystitis infections. According to Dr. Jackie McGroarty of Toronto General Hospital, nonoxynol-9™, the active component of these creams (and incidentally, the ingredient recommended to protect against the AIDS virus), promotes the growth of E. coli (a bacteria that causes cystitis) and candida albicans. At the same time, the chemical kills lactobaccilli which are found in large numbers in the vagina and which are thought to provide protection against the growth of disease-causing microorganisms.

CHAPTER SEVEN

PARASITES,
THE FORGOTTEN DIAGNOSIS

Susan K. went to her doctor in early January because she had had diarrhea and vomiting with low grade fever for three days. She thought perhaps she had an intestinal virus and that her doctor could at least prescribe something to relieve her symptoms. Her doctor asked her if she had just returned from the tropics. "No," she said, "but I did visit Colorado over the holidays."

Susan's doctor ordered a stool culture and, to her surprise, found that she had a parasite called Giardia Lamblia. He prescribed a course of Flagyl, and following that, supplements to encourage the regrowth of intestinal flora. Susan was back to normal within two weeks.

Most Americans, including many physicians, tend to consider intestinal parasites a problem indigenous to poor, underdeveloped countries. Diseases caused by organisms with names like Entamoeba Hystolitica or Giardia Lamblia seem to suggest tropical and unsanitary origins. Of course, those conditions do appear most frequently in underdeveloped countries where sanitation is lacking.

However, as Susan's doctor was aware, there are many places in the U.S. where parasites abound. For instance, many mountainous areas, where wild animals are urinating into the streams, become areas of giardiasis contamination.

Despite our beliefs about parasites, they have no respect for socio-economic status. Because the signs and symptoms of intestinal parasitic infections are often vague, and because many physicians in this country are not familiar with them, a patient may endure discomfort for weeks or months before the proper diagnosis is made.

Since the treatment of such illnesses is now much more effective than ever before, it pays to know something about these problems.

This chapter will give you information on when to suspect parasites as the cause of your symptoms. And, more important, it tells you how to prevent them.

Parasites are able to take advantage of a weakened immune system to spread throughout the body, combining with other viruses and yeast cells. It is important to realize that CFIDS patients will not improve without first excluding parasites as the cause of symptoms, and then treating existing parasites.

Blastocystis hominis, cryptosporidium and *endolimax nina* are considered to be non-pathogenic (non-disease-causing) by most mainstream doctors. But in someone whose immune system is already suppressed, even these parasites can spell trouble. Thirty years ago, Giardia was considered a harmless parasite in humans. The same misconception is still true with Blastocystis hominis.

In a Saudi Arabian study, undertaken over two years and involving 12,136 patients, research pathologists concluded that "B. hominis should be considered as a causative agent of human disease in patient, with recurrent symptoms, especially when the parasite is present in large numbers in fecal specimens in the absence of other known pathogens. We have discontinued to consider B. hominis as non-pathogenic." (Ref. #1)

Symptoms of Parasitic Infection

Many times, parasitic infections cause nonspecific, generalized symptoms. Physicians should consider the possibility of parasitic infection if their patients' symptoms persist after treatment for viral diseases or candida. For instance, if a patient has been adequately treated for yeast overgrowth and still experiences persistent gas, bloating and allergic reactions to foodstuffs which do not cause yeast growth, there is a possibility of parasitosis.

Leo Galland, M.D., and three colleagues demonstrated in 1990 that 61 patients out of 218 suffering from chronic fatigue were infected with Giardia. Treatment for giardiasis produced a complete cure of fatigue in 13 out of 48 patients, marked improvement in 21 out of 48 patients and some benefit in 8 out of 48 patients. (2)

Parasites can be present even without specific symptoms or a positive lab test. In fact, 50% of infected patients have no symptoms at all. The following nonspecific symptoms may suggest the presence of parasites:

* Foul-smelling intestinal gas, worse in the afternoon and evening.
* A change in bowel habits, sometimes gradual, over a period of weeks or months. This is the most common symptom.
* Soft or watery bowel movements, or, paradoxically, constipation. As time goes on, severe constipation is a more likely development.
* Abdominal cramps and increased rumbling and gurgling in the abdomen, unrelated to hunger and food intake.
* Weight loss in spite of ravenous appetite.
* Itching around the anus, particularly at night when the female pinworms crawl out of the rectum to lay their eggs under the skin.
* Food allergies, especially to foods that will not feed yeast cells (rice or corn, for example).
* A pneumonia-like illness, with cough, wheezing and fever, as well as a swelling of the liver. In this case, the cause is roundworms.
* Some relief experienced after eating some food.
* For women, sore and swollen breasts not related to the menstrual cycle.
* Depression.
* Incomplete bowel movements.
* Chest pain, heartburn or heart pain.
* Extreme bloating. This is one of the most common symptoms.

As you can see, none of these symptoms is **the** isolated symptom of a parasitic infection.   But because of the similarity in symptoms, parasitic infection should be ruled out with every immune-suppressed patient. The combination of clinical symptoms and the most reliable lab tests available will yield the correct diagnosis.

Diagnosis of Parasitic Infection

Stool Cultures

Until recently, diagnosis of parasitic infection was made through repeated stool cultures (three days in a row) by a laboratory experienced in detecting parasites. However, the proper diagnosis was often missed because of falsely negative lab tests. Parasites were found in only 25% of these cases. Parasites tend to dig into the intestinal lining, so it is often unlikely they will be isolated in small stool samples. A three-day stool sample is more accurate, since it increases the chances of finding parasites, but still falls short of the best method. By using the purged stool test, more pieces of the diagnostic puzzle can be found.

Capturing Eggs

Tapeworms are best diagnosed by finding eggs in the stool or around the anus. Pinworms are best detected by examining the anal area for tiny white worms at night about two hours after the sufferer goes to bed. Cellophane tape placed around the anal opening in the morning can pick up the eggs which are visible only under a microscope.

Purged Stool Test

By far the best parasite test is the purged stool test, produced by Dowell Laboratory, of Mesa, Arizona. (Tel. 602-964-7151) As with regular stool tests, patients take a stool kit home with them. Three days before the test, the patient has to avoid eating red meat, and for one day before, must avoid all red fruit and vegetable juices. On the morning of the test, which is done in the privacy of each patient's home, the patient has no breakfast. In the stool kit is a liquid laxative (unfortunately salty tasting, but very effective). Half of this laxative is swallowed and within two hours, 80% of the patients will have at least six very loose bowel movements. It is the sixth stool sample that will be returned in the little bottle provided. About 20% of the patients, usually those with a history of severe blockage in the gastrointestinal tract, may take several more hours to accomplish their task. A loose stool is imperative for a reliable reading. A half-formed stool can produce false negative results.

In the table below, you will see an example of stool test results as provided by Dowell Lab. Interpretation of the test is easily done by the doctor and even you, the patient. It takes only about 30 minutes to perform this test in the lab. Results can be available within five working days. It will help you to interpret your own purged stool. This test is also useful in detecting monilia (candida) or yeast overgrowth, especially when it is abundant.

TABLE 4

**EXAMPLE OF A PURGED STOOL TEST
AND HOW TO READ IT**

Color: yellow-orange: has a lot to do with cleansing
Consistency: watery (unless the stool is watery, the stool is not purged)
Occult (hidden) blood: 4+: pathogenic; lower/upper GI indicated; up to 2+ normal.
Mucus: trace amounts (sometimes excessive mucus is present)
Bacteria: essentially absent (lack of friendly bacteria)
Yeast: abundant monilia (candida): pathogenic
PMN (Polymorfonuclear cells - white blood cells): occasional (indicative of white blood cells, present for your defense)
Red blood cells: none seen; has to be under 2/hdf (in the microscopic field viewed)
Ova (eggs): negative, for instance, ova of Ascaris
Parasites: Giardia lamblia (cysts): pathogenic; immature forms (cysts) will require long-term treatment
Other: Bile stained: indicates pancreatic deficiency

The above is a typical example of a purged stool test result. As is seen in the example, it is common to have abundant yeast and parasites at the same time. Failure to treat parasites would keep the yeast alive, and symptoms of CFIDS, for instance, would not go away.

Bueno-Parish Test

Another test also performed to detect amebiasis is the Bueno-Parish test, in which the doctor or nurse will take a rectal swab using a small rectal speculum. This method is certainly more accurate than the regular stool cultures performed. However, the swab requires expertise and therefore tends to be a little more unreliable than the purged stool test. But the Bueno-Parish test is definitely a good alternative for patients who cannot handle the purged stool kit laxative, either because of its salty taste, hypersensitivity to medication, or heightened weakness and dehydration.

Parasitic Panel

Another alternative is a parasitic panel, a blood test performed by ITL, in which antibodies to entamoeba histolytica, Giardia lamblia and toxoplasma gondii are measured. Also, be aware of parasites if the eosinophils (another type of white blood cell) are out of the normal range, i.e., increased.

Common Parasites and Their Treatments

If you suspect, from the symptoms already outlined in this chapter, that you have parasites, you may want to mention your suspicions to your doctor. When your immume system is suppressed, parasites and yeast can easily invade your body, further taxing your weakened defense system.

Since parasites are so prevalent, it's a good idea to know a little about their transmission. If you know this, you can take simple hygienic precautions to avoid infection. This section provides a description of the most common types.

Table 5 on the next page illustrates the different possible parasites present in human beings.

Roundworms

More than a million Americans are believed to harbor the giant roundworm, Ascaris Lumbricoides, which may reach 14 inches in length. It is relatively common in the southern United States, but can also be found in other areas.

It is contracted by ingesting the eggs of the worm, when eating meat, or from pet dogs or cats. More than 80% of the puppies born in this country are infected with roundworm. Children who play with these infected animals and who put their hands in their mouths are susceptible to infection. Therefore, the best way to avoid contracting this parasite is to take your puppy or kitten to the vet for treatment at the age of three weeks.

If you have roundworms, the therapy is relatively simple. You can take six **Vermox tabs,** two a day for three days in a row. Make sure you have an excellent bowel movement the third day after taking the last dose (an enema might be useful). Often, when symptoms persist, the therapeutic trial has to be repeated one week later.

TABLE 5

COMMON PARASITES FOUND
IN PURGED STOOL

Family	Purged Stool Exam	Significance
Sarcodina	Endolimax Nana	Commensal (non-pathogenic)
	Entameba Coli	Commensal (except children)
	Entameba Histolytica	pathogenic/carcinogenic
Mastigophera	Giardia lamblia	Pathogenic
	Trichomonas hominis	Commensal (except children)
Sporozoa	Cryptosporidium	Semi-pathogen, self-limiting, except in immune impaired patients; mold-related
Nematoda	Ascaris Lumbric. (round worm)	Pathogenic
	Enterobius Vern.	Pathogenic
	Trichuris Trichura	Pathogenic
Cestoda	Taenia	Pathogenic (pork/beef)
Blastocystis hominis		Pathogenic in immune suppressed patients

Tapeworms

You can get tapeworms by ingesting raw or inadequately cooked beef, pork, or fish that is contaminated with tapeworm eggs. The beef tapeworm is common in the United States, while the pork tapeworm is prevalent in Asia and Eastern Europe. Fish tapeworms are found in fresh-water fish in Scandinavia, Japan, Canada and Florida. The best prevention is to avoid raw and uncooked meat and fish. The best medical treatment is Yomesan, two grams daily for seven days. It is advisable to take a purge after this treatment.

Pinworms

Some 20 million Americans, most of them children between the ages of two and four, are suffering from these small (half-inch-long) parasites. The parasite is spread by contact with infected clothing, bedding and toys, and by contact with other infected children, who may carry the eggs under their fingernails and spread them to others directly.

The best treatment is to take two tablets of Vermox daily for three days. There are chewable tablets available for children. An alternative is Mintezol chewable tablets, two doses daily for two days.

Amoebiasis Giardiasis and Shigellosis

Giardiasis has now reached almost epidemic proportions. This protozoan infection is now known to be spreading throughout the United States. It has caused community-wide outbreaks in some places where the water supply is chlorinated but not filtered. Giardia also infects beavers and dogs, who may contaminate reservoirs with their feces. It is also a common cause of traveler's diarrhea, as with Susan K.

Because they are extremely hardy, the giardia parasites are difficult and expensive to remove from a contaminated water supply. Giardiasis is especially prevalent in mountain areas because the cysts survive best in cold water. They can be killed by adding chlorine and letting the water sit for a long time, or by using a special filtering system. To prevent possible infection, you should not drink the water at mountain restaurants and you should always bring your own bottled water for drinking. If you do a lot of camping and traveling in mountain areas, you should be on the alert for a pure water supply. Check with the local authorities, who do regular testing of the mountainous water supply.

Another transmission method has been recently identified in urban areas. It has been shown that this infection can be transmitted during sex, especially among the gay population, and it is this group that is presently at risk. The cysts of Entamoeba Hystolitica and Giardia Lamblia can retain their infectivity for considerable periods of time outside the human host. Consequently, any type of sexual activity that includes anal-oral contact is a potential source of infection.

Entamoeba Hystolitica

Entamoeba Hystolitica is the parasite that causes amebiasis, more commonly known as amebic dysentery. It is found in every country in the world, though its effects are more severe in warmer climates. It travels with enormous speed through the intestines. Amebas can live only a short time outside the host's body. In their dormant form, however, amebas become all-but-impermeable cysts that are amazingly resistant to the disinfectant chlorine and to extreme temperatures. These cysts can survive outside the body for a long time before being passed in stools for years by carriers who have a chronic, asymptomatic form of the disease. In fact, the greatest danger is that some carriers never develop symptoms! Unfortunately, an amebiasis victim with no symptoms is just as contagious as one in excruciating pain.

According to UNICEF, more than two billion people are threatened by amebiasis in developing countries. Because of a lack of sanitary facilities and running water, many people die from its effects.

You may be thinking, "But I don't visit exotic countries. I don't need to worry about this." But even in the U.S., as many as 200,000 gay men may be afflicted with this disease.

Even if you are not gay or have not traveled to these exotic areas, you can still have been exposed, just by eating in restaurants. Recent immigrants to the U.S. often seek jobs in restaurant kitchens, because of low entry-level pay and the absence of immigration requirements. Some immigrants from third world countries may be asymptomatic carriers of amebiasis. As carriers, they are just as contagious as those with full-blown symptoms. So if kitchen workers are not fastidious about cleanliness, especially hand-washing, the disease can be spread to customers.

One step forward would be greater involvement by state health departments. An excellent step would be to require a stool examination as a condition of employment from all employees that handle or serve food to the public in schools, restaurants, cafeterias or grocery stores. If people are reluctant to have the stool test, a blood test is fairly accurate to at least detect the carriers of cysts.

Since the symptoms of amebiasis are generalized, some people affected do not consult their doctors. A person who has bloating, gas or loose stools might just say, "I ate too much," or, "I drank too much coffee or alcohol." And remember, these symptoms come and go. So few patients with the parasitic disease will be diagnosed, and because of the inaccuracy of regular stool tests, still fewer will be treated.

Studies done by the Department of Health and the Gay Men's Health Project in New York City, showed that 30% of randomly selected individuals harbored protozoal organisms, primarily Entamoeba Hystolitica and G. Lamblia. Another study was done at the Cornell Medical Center, and again selection was limited to volunteering gay patients. The statistics were similar: almost 40% of the patients were infected with amoebas. We know that in healthy individuals, amebiasis is usually not a morbid disease. Immature amebas migrate to the large intestines, and live there without causing any symptoms. However, if a patient's immune system is already suppressed from other conditions, such as CFIDS, candida and other Herpes Simplex viruses, wouldn't it be better to eliminate any further taxes on the system?

* Treatment: At this point, Flagyl is the medically accepted remedy for amebiasis. Unfortunately, its side effects can be considerable. It causes headaches, nausea, depression, disorientation and attacks of vertigo. Sometimes patients have to repeat several rounds of Flagyl before the amebas are eradicated. Even more unfortunate is that Flagyl favors growth of yeast. Since most parasite carriers will also suffer from yeast (remember these two are like family members supporting each other and housed in the same environment), Flagyl makes most of these patients so ill they have to stop taking Flagyl after a couple of days. There are natural alternatives are available, discussed at the end of this chapter.

Giardia Lamblia

The fresh, fast-flowing waters of the mountainous areas of North America are no longer as inviting as they used to be. Skiing or backpacking vacations in the Rocky Mountains and parts of New England, where the water is derived mainly from surface sources, may be marred by a diarrheal illness; the agent most likely to be responsible is the protozoan intestinal parasite, Giardia Lamblia. However, unlike the acute bacterial diarrhea common to travelers in the tropics, the diarrhea resulting from G. Lamblia is not likely to spoil a patient's holidays. Symptoms usually do not begin for a week or more after ingestion of contaminated water or food, by which time the patients are usually back home. Returning to work, however, may be another experience altogether.

G. Lamblia is presently one of the most frequently identifiable causes of water-borne diarrhea in the United States. The main stumbling block in the management of Giardiasis is the diagnosis. A number of cases are missed in the early stages because of a low index of suspicion by the physician; and even if detected, Giardia is frequently considered a harmless organism in the human gastrointestinal tract.

It was not until 1965, during an outbreak in Aspen, Colorado, that water supplies were suspected as the source of Giardiasis. We now know that the danger of Giardiasis exists in all areas where surface waters may be contaminated or where there is inadequate treatment of main water supplies. This can occur in remote, wilderness areas as well as in large urban centers.

Giardiasis can also be spread by uncooked contaminated foods. Some people may be more susceptible to Giardiasis than others. People living in areas where surface waters are contaminated usually do not contract the disease, probably because they have become immune. There is also some evidence that genetic factors might play a role. For example, it seems that people with type A blood are more likely to get Giardiasis than people with other blood types. Gastrectomy (removal of part of or the whole stomach) and achlorhydria (absence of hydrochloric acid) in adults are predisposing factors to an increased susceptibility to developing symptomatic Giardiasis, because the gastric acid barrier is missing.

The symptoms are mainly those described on pages 83 and 84. Again it is important to remember that 20% to 50% of those who excrete Giardia cysts have no symptoms. The acute stage lasts from a few days to three weeks. Especially foul-smelling stools, absence of blood and mucus in the stools, and excessive foul flatulence in association with marked distention are features more characteristic of Giardiasis.

* Diagnosis: A routine question for any patient with protracted diarrhea (lasting for more than seven days) should be, "Where have you been?" If the patient hasn't been traveling, the physicians should inquire about possible episodes of direct or indirect oral-The accurate test is usually the purged stool test. If, at the end, Giardiasis is strongly suspected but tests are negative, an empiric therapeutic trial is worthwhile.

Treatment for Giardia and E. *Histolytica: Here is a list of the available drugs, all of which should be avoided during pregnancy!*

-Atabrine (Quinacrine) is the one most used. Cure rates of about 80% can be expected. But adverse reactions such as nausea, vomiting, urticaria (an itchy rash) and a drug-induced, short-term psychosis, together with the relatively long treatment (at least seven days), make it considerably less desirable than newer drugs. The normal dose is 100 mg three times a day for seven days.

-Flagyl (Metronidazole), although not approved by the FDA for this indication, is the treatment of choice especially in developing countries. It is given as a single 2g dose on three successive days. Lack of appetite, nausea, abdominal pain and diarrhea are possible. One drawback is that it can stimulate the overgrowth of yeast.

-Tinidazole is widely used in other parts of the world. It is highly effective as a single dose of 2g. It is available in suppository form for children.

Although all these agents are rather effective, none of them is ideal. (3) A safe, easily tolerated drug or supplement, which is effective as a single dose, is clearly needed.

Natural Therapy for Parasites

Because of the side-effects of all the above medications, I prefer the natural available products as a first-line therapeutic approach.

A Medication Devoid of Side Effects

While black walnut and garlic have been proven to be effective in the battle against parasites, I prefer the combination of a **grapefruit seed extract (Paramycrocidin)** and another herbal product, **Artemesia annua,** taken in a dose of 1,000 mg t.i.d. for at least 60 days. Follow-up purged stool cultures have shown this treatment to be effective. There are hardly any side effects. The medication is best taken with food since it can be rather hard on the stomach. CFIDS patients suffering from parasitosis will see improvement from the first days on. One of the first corrections is the formation of more voluminous bowel movements instead of the loose or hardened stools these patients suffer from. Other signs of a correct diagnosis and successful therapy will be the disappearance of food sensitivities and bloating. Once the symptoms have cleared and stool cultures show no more parasites, acidophilus should be added in order to prevent recurrence of parasites.

Other Natural Products

Other useful natural products which can be used against parasites include papaya seeds (used extensively in Mexico), pumpkin seeds (a diuretic, but also useful as an anthelminthic), and wormseed (also known as Jerusalem artichoke).

Prevention is the Key

Because there is no single totally effective medication that will eradicate parasitic infection, prevention is the ideal medicine. Here are some tips:

1. Continue your treatment until all of your family members have been tested (and treated, when necessary).

2. If you eat in restaurants, avoid raw foods, such as salads and sushi. The safest bet is to eat well-cooked foods.

3. At home, peel all your vegetables and soak them in water and vinegar (mixed 1:1) for 15 minutes.

4. As with any immuno-suppressed condition, your ultimate goal is to strengthen your immune system, so exposure to common parasites will not make you ill.

5. When you travel, follow these rules:

* Don't drink the water unless it has been boiled or bottled.
* Don't eat fruit unless it has been peeled.
* Avoid salads, cold platters, pastries, custards, ice, mayonnaise and uncooked or undercooked meat.
* Don't use tap water in bathrooms to brush your teeth.
* Don't swallow water when taking a bath.
* Don't swim in polluted water.
* Don't drink water that is not carbonated. (Carbonation makes it harder for bacteria to survive.)
* Avoid using Pepto-Bismol ™ as a preventative. It contains aspirin and acts as a blood thinner. It can keep toxins in the body, rather than excreting them. You are much better taking psyllium husk and daily doses of acidophilus.
* Avoid dehydration if you do get an attack of traveler's diarrhea. You can accomplish this by drinking a lot of fluids, rice water, and avoiding coffee and tea (caffeine is a diuretic and will cause you to lose fluids.) Eat some saltine crackers or dry toast.

Exposure to parasites is no longer the sole province of the world traveler. People in urban environments need to practice good preventive techniques and be on the alert for symptoms which If you suffer from candida, CFIDS, AIDS or herpes simplex viruses, ask your doctor to look for parasites. If your physician does not suggest the possibility, you can ask for a stool test. Your immune system will thank you for the rest of your life.

In the next chapter, we cover the treatments for viral and yeast infections. We have seen in Chapters Six and Seven how important it is not to unwittingly feed micro-organisms like yeast and parasites. Food choices and eating habits are important to us all, but especially so for any any CFIDS or immuno-suppressed patient.

The next chapter deals with the most serious of the immune system disorders: AIDS, or Acquired Immune Deficiency Syndrome.

REFERENCES
(1). "Clinical Significance of Blastocystis Hominis," Hussain Qadri, G.A. Al-Okaili, and F. Al-Dayel, Department of Pathology, King Faisal Hospital and Research Centre, Saudi Arabia; *Journal of Clinical Microbiology*, Vol. 27, No. 11, November, 1989, pp. 2407-2409.
(2). "Giardia lamblia Infection as a Cause of Chronic Fatigue", Leo Galland MD, Marty Lee PhD, Herman Bueno MD, C. Heimowitz MS, Meadowlands Clinical Laboratory, Rutherford, NJ 07070; *Journal of Nutritional Medicine* (1990) 1, 27-31
(3). "Effect of Twenty-three Chemotherapeutic Agents on the Adherence and Growth of Giardia lamblia in Vitro", Crouch, Seow and Thong; Dept. of Pathology, Mater Hospital, University of Queensland, South Brisbane, Australia 4101; *Transactions of the Royal Society of Tropical Medicine and Hygiene* (1986) 80, 893-896.

Other Useful References:
(1). "Chronic Giardiasis: Studies on Drug Sensitivity, Toxin Production and Host Immune Response," Philip Smith, et al.; Laboratory of Parasitic Diseases, Bethesda, Maryland; *Gastroenterology*, Vol. 83; 1982; pages 797-803.
(2). "Chemotherapy in Giardisis: Clinical Responses and In Vitro Drug Sensitivity of Human Isolates in Axenic Cultures," Peter McIntyre, M.B., B.S., et al., Department of Child Health, University of Queensland, Australia; *Journal of Pediatrics*, Vol. 108, No. 6, June, 1986; pages 1005-1009.
(3) "In Vitro Response of Blastocystis Hominis to Antiprotozoal Drugs," Charles Zierdt, et al., Department of Clinical Pathology, Bethesda, Maryland, *Journal of Protozool*, Vol 30, No. 2; 1983, pages 332-334.

CHAPTER EIGHT

AIDS: IS THERE A LINK WITH OTHER IMMUNE-SUPPRESSED CONDITIONS?

Acquired Immune Deficiency Syndrome (AIDS) is increasingly being seen as a consuming global problem. Although the worst is happening in Africa and other third world nations, the effects of this disease on our own economic and social structure will be massive, and last well into the 21st Century.

The HIV virus is especially virulent, capable of taking over the defense system and turning it against itself. Because of its long latency period (anywhere from six months to several years), it is difficult to predict the numbers of those who will be ultimately affected. Cure is still off in the future. So what remains for those at risk is to develop safe sex practices, build up the immune system, and be alert to other invaders that may weaken the body's defenses.

Keep in mind that herpes and candidiasis, both immune-suppressed conditions, run on the same "freeway" as AIDS. Chronic Epstein Barr virus, the herpes simplex viruses, and some of the retroviruses, such as HTLV-2, are at the entrance to this "freeway," putting in motion a chain of events that leads to a continuously suppressed immune system. And as you saw in Chapter Three, an immune system under continuous assault will eventually break down. The body can become more vulnerable to attack when exposed to AIDS.

AIDS is no longer a complete mystery to medical scientists, as it was in the early 1980's when the syndrome began claiming lives in large numbers. What this chapter describes are the spreading mechanisms of the AIDS virus, the co-factors which make people more vulnerable to it, preventive measures to protect oneself, and recommendations for building immunity against it.

How the Virus Works

The invader is tiny, about 1/16,000th the size of a pinhead. Its structure is very basic: a double-layered shell of proteins around a nucleus of RNA, or ribonucleic acid. The virus is present in the blood and bodily fluids, and is transmitted via those fluids when there is direct contact, as in sexual intercourse, or from the placenta of an infected mother to her baby. As in the case with any invasion, the immune system is alerted at the moment of intrusion and sends an array of cells to deal with this threat. But herein lies the danger. The AIDS virus seems to ignore most of the body's defender cells. It zooms in on the receptor, found on the surface of the "General" of the immune system, the helper T cell. It fits on the receptor like the perfect key into a lock, and the door to our most sensitive and valuable system opens wide. The virus penetrates the cell membrane, stripping away the cell's protective shell in the process. Within half an hour, the virus and its enzyme are floating in the cytoplasm, the fluid interior of the cell.

With the help of its enzyme, the AIDS virus then converts its RNA into DNA (double-stranded deoxyribonucleic acid), the master molecule of life. The DNA penetrates the cell nucleus and inserts itself into a chromosome. This process activates a new cellular machinery, directed at producing more of these deadly viruses. Eventually the cell swells and dies, releasing a new flood of viruses to attack other cells, including more helper T cells and macrophages. The immune system, stripped of its crucial defenders, the T cells, therefore responds inadequately to attacks by other infectious agents. This is the moment when exotic and opportunistic bacteria and viruses attack the body. Having reached this point, it is only a matter of time: the AIDS victim usually succumbs to these other infections.

Theories about the Origin of AIDS

It is now generally accepted by the medical community that HIV is the cause of AIDS. Ordinarily, a person is at risk until he or she forms antibodies against a virus. Yet with AIDS — if we accept that HIV is the cause — the disease progresses, paradoxically, after antibodies have been formed. The fact that the disease progresses in the face of intact immunity could suggest that HIV is not the culprit. It may well be that blood containing the HIV virus includes also whatever agent it is that actually causes the disease. It may be worthwhile to examine the various other theories about the origin of AIDS in order to expand our understanding of the epidemic. I emphasize that all of them are speculative and only theories, with the most basic questions unanswered.

Green Monkey Transference Theory

This theory is probably the most popular one. A virus called STLV-3, known to cause a mild AIDS-like disease, was discovered in green monkeys. In order for human beings to come into contact with the virus, they either have to be bitten by the green monkey or have monkey blood spilled into human sores and cuts. However, neither of these transferring methods explains the explosion of AIDS seen in Africa. The number of people affected by AIDS surpasses by a wide margin the estimate based on the transference theory. Nevertheless, certain scientists hold to this theory, claiming that the virus underwent a mutation in these monkeys several years ago. However, the AIDS virus is more rapidly mutating than any animal virus yet studied.

African Swine Fever Theory

Another theory suggests a relationship to African Swine Fever (ASF), a deadly and rapidly transmitted disease spread among pigs — and to humans — by ticks. Swine-fever pigs exhibit symptoms similar to those of AIDS and ARC patients, specifically lesions common to victims of Kaposi's sarcoma. Researchers noticed that wherever there was a concentration of swine fever, there was a concentration of AIDS. That includes the Florida outbreak of ASF between 1979 and 1983, which may have been brought there by Haitian boat people and their livestock.

However, the mainstream medical community maintains that ASF is not a disease that can harm man. The CDC tried to replicate previous conclusive studies, but found "no positive evidence." Nevertheless, many other scientists are critical of these conclusions and continue to investigate a possible connection.

Smallpox Vaccine Theory

This theory was first published in the London Times in May, 1987. The reported investigation indicated that a popular smallpox vaccine was spreading the epidemic. The World Health Organization categorically denies this. The theory would, however, provide a possible explanation for the highest incidence in Central African states, since it corresponds with the most intense smallpox immunization program.

How Was AIDS Spread?

How did this nightmare enter the United States? What happened, and why has the epidemic spread so far? Doctors initially traced the first cases back to 1979. However, in 1987 researchers jolted the medical community with evidence that the disease may have made its first appearance in the United States almost 15 years earlier. It was the story of a young black man, 16 years old, who showed up at the St. Louis City Hospital with chronic genital swelling. Researchers found chlamydia, a genital bacterial infection common in sexually active persons. But what was strange was that he did not respond to routine therapy. His muscles wasted away, and he died shortly thereafter, leaving the medical community mystified. In the hope that medical advances might someday solve this mystery, his blood was frozen. In 1987, his blood tested positive for the AIDS virus.

What we can conclude from this is that the history of AIDS in the U.S. may have a much longer prologue than was once suspected. It probably was around for a long time but just wasn't recognized. It certainly predates the case of the Canadian flight attendant, Gaetan Dugas, who for a long time was considered "Patient Zero," since he was the key transmitter, responsible for the first recorded cluster of AIDS patients. Traveling extensively, Dugas was able to spread the disease to different corners of the country, making it difficult at first for scientists to link all these cases. However, his name kept popping up, and it was this that put researchers on the right track. The links bore out fears about the virus having a long latency period. For instance, some of the victims did not show symptoms until months after Dugas had spent the weekend with them. Since the AIDS virus was not epidemic in 1969 (when Robert R., the St. Louis teenager, was diagnosed) it is possible that it mutated and became more virulent in the 1970s.

What we do know is that AIDS is spread through exchange of bodily fluids, and through contact with blood and blood products. The primary avenues of infection are sexual contact (exchange of bodily fluids) and transfusions (with infected blood and blood products).

Who Is At Greatest Risk?

What is the number of actual AIDS cases at this point? The Centers for Disease Control (CDC) states that of the 160,000 cases of AIDS reported in the U.S. since 1981, 100,000 patients died by the end of 1990. The death toll is climbing, and it is projected that in the next three years as many as 200,000 more Americans will die of AIDS. The CDC also estimates that one million Americans are already infected with the AIDS virus. The World Health Organization (WHO) estimates that there are more than 300,000 cases of AIDS worldwide and about 10 million people infected with the AIDS virus. Of these 10 million, WHO estimates, an additional three million women and children will die of AIDS. In major American and European cities, AIDS has become the leading cause of death for women aged 20 to 40. But in places like Africa, WHO suspects an underdiagnosing of AIDS because of inaccurate reporting systems.

How many people are at risk? The world's population now is five billion, with about 130 million births and 50 million deaths each year.

The estimated 10 million infected people represent a small minority at risk of contracting AIDS. Those at highest risk fall into four main groups:

* Sexually transmitted group (mainly homosexuals and bisexuals, but also heterosexual partners of intravenous drug users)
* Intravenous drug users group
* Blood transfusion group
* Newborn group
* Sexually transmitted group

The estimated 105 million people worldwide who develop sexually transmitted diseases such as syphilis, gonorrhea or herpes are more likely to be exposed to other sexually transmitted diseases, including AIDS. In fact, the concomitant presence of herpes, syphilis, and also hepatitis B will decrease the strength of the immune system enough to bring these victims into a group more likely to contract AIDS upon contact with the AIDS virus.

There is another condition reaching epidemic proportions: yeast infections, part of the CFIDS pandemic. We have already discussed how this widespread problem, often unrecognized and untreated, can wreak havoc with the immune system, giving the AIDS virus a good opportunity to roam through a weakened immune system. Those high levels of exposure to the other viruses and yeast cells apparently cause a "chronically activated immune state," which may increase vulnerability to AIDS. These facts might be clues as to why certain people seem to be less susceptible than others and why sex partners of some AIDS patients remain free of infection.

Homosexuals were the first community to be identified in the spreading of this syndrome. The risk factors include multiple sex partners and the practice of receptive anal intercourse. Sexually transmitted disease is often quite common. What we now know about the immune system suggests that these men, contracting recurrent sexually-transmitted diseases, had more stress on their immune systems, leaving them at higher risk for developing AIDS.

Homosexuals form a very well-known group, but very little is known about the numbers and habits of bisexuals. Bisexuals are most likely conduits for the spread of AIDS to heterosexuals, who may bed them or, as often happens, marry them, never suspecting that their partners are leading a dangerous double love-life.

It is difficult for public health officials to pinpoint the extent of infection in the population. Heterosexual contact is the main route of transmission in Africa. It isn't here in the United States, where gays, bisexuals and intravenous-drug users make up the vast majority of AIDS victims. Only four percent of the 35,000 known cases in 1989 are attributed to heterosexual contact, and this percentage has remained the same for nearly a decade.

Because it can take eight years or more from the time of infection to develop AIDS, looking at current victims only tells us what was happening years ago. To discover whether there is a "breakout" into the heterosexual majority, you have to look at who is now infected, not who has already developed the disease. The government is planning a national survey to determine the prevalence of the virus. Another study, planned on the advice of former Surgeon General C. Everett Koop, is HIV testing in a major college to determine the prevalence of AIDS among adolescents. But both studies will only tell us how far the AIDS epidemic has spread, not how *fast* it is spreading.

So far, we are not in for a rapid sweep into the heterosexual population, as has occurred in Africa. Africa, with its different cultural norms, sometimes polygamous societies, poor public health picture and assorted sexual diseases, is still quite different. Unfortunately, an "African-style" AIDS explosion is not the only thing to worry about. The CDC never predicted a quick outbreak, only a slow expansion until, by 1992, nine percent of the 270,000 dead AIDS victims (hardly a small health problem) will be heterosexuals who are not drug users. Studies show that "only" 36 percent of California women who were frequent sex partners of AIDS victims got the virus. But is that encouraging? I think that more than one out of three is rather high. So it remains to be seen whether a heterosexual explosion of AIDS might occur in the future.

An interesting study to determine the odds of getting AIDS from a single act of heterosexual intercourse was published in the April, 1988 *Journal of the American Medical Association*. Doctors Norman Hearst and Stephen Hulley, epidemiologists at the University of California at San Francisco Medical School, estimated that the chance of catching the AIDS virus from a single act of heterosexual intercourse with a low-risk partner is one in five billion if a condom is used. The risk rises to one in 500 if the partner is known to be infected and no condom is used. Then there is the middle group: one-time sex with someone who is not in a high-risk group but whose infection state is unknown. The risk of infection here is one in five million without a condom.

* Intravenous drug users group

Because drug addicts often share needles, or use dirty or contaminated syringes to inject their drugs, this is one of the largest group of infected individuals. HIV-positive drug users then infect their sexual partners. If their wives become pregnant, then their children are also unfortunately affected. It is difficult to estimate the exact number of regular intravenous-drug users in the world. New York, with its vast population of drug users, has been hit the hardest. Intravenous drug users also tend to neglect every other aspect of their health. With irregular and often unhealthy eating habits, no exercise and emotional instability due to the precarious lifestyle, their defenses may be especially easy to penetrate.

* Blood transfusion group

Many people with chronic illness rely on blood transfusion on a regular basis for survival. Unbeknownst to medical science, the HIV virus was present in the general population before 1981, when the first cluster of disease was identified. Before that time, there was no procedure for testing donated blood for the virus, because the virus was not yet known. Unfortunately, millions of people received transfusions between 1978 and 1985. According to one estimate, the risk of contracting AIDS from blood transfusions is one in 250,000. Of course, this is small consolation for those who received transfusions to save their lives and got a deadly disease instead.

How big is the problem so far? Almost one thousand transfusion-associated cases were recorded through 1990. Nearly half of these incidents were in New York or California. Infants, who receive less than two percent of all transfusions, nevertheless represent 10 percent of transfusion-related cases of AIDS. However, the CDC estimates that as many as 12,000 of the 34 million who received blood before it was screened in 1984 may have been infected. It was recommended that all these transfusion recipients should be tested for the virus. The study on which the recommendation was based — a study done at New York City's Sloan-Kettering Memorial Center — caused panic among the population who flooded telephone lines at blood centers. Health officials estimate that one in every 2,500 units of blood was contaminated.

Since 1984, however, elimination of HIV in blood transfusions by antibody screening has drastically reduced the number of AIDS cases resulting from transfusions. Also, with the present insecurities about the blood supply, candidates for scheduled and elective surgeries either donate their own blood (autologous transfusions) or receive it from family members (directed transfusions), increasing the safety for these patients.

* Newborn group

Because the baby gets its blood supply directly from the mother during pregnancy, the risk that an infected woman will infect her baby is probably high, yet not clearly determined. According to the CDC, about 620 cases of pediatric AIDS have been documented since doctors identified the syndrome in 1983; two thirds of those patients have died. While at this moment it is estimated that about 2,000 children in the nation are sick with HIV infection, the total expected number in 1991 of children showing symptoms of AIDS infection will be between 10,000 and 20,000.

Who will care for them? It is a fact that nearly all of them are or will be born into poor families where drug abuse is rampant. However, this is one class of HIV-infected people we can protect today: next year's infected newborns are not yet conceived.

Sub-groups of Transmitters

We just discussed the four main groups of AIDS transmitters. Some claim that there are four additional routes for AIDS to be transmitted:

* Through non-sexual contact with AIDS-contaminated blood
* Through artificial insemination
* From mosquito bites
* From organ transplants

Thousands of health workers have reported pricking themselves with needles used on AIDS victims, yet the incidence of AIDS among them is exceptionally low. What these small numbers of cases should teach us is the need for extreme caution. Whenever care givers come into contact with body fluids of AIDS patients, they should wear gloves, goggles and masks. The cases of three female health workers were the first incidence of transmission of the virus reported in victims *without* a needle prick. But all these women had breaks in their skin that could have allowed the virus to enter. Consequently, the risk to health workers is still very low. Until 1990, it was doctors and other health care workers who feared being infected by patients, and many doctors called for mandatory testing of patients. There was little concern about transmitting the AIDS virus from infected doctors to patients. But the summer of 1990 changed all that. The CDC in Atlanta reported that a Florida dentist, Dr. Acer, apparently transmitted the AIDS virus to one of his patients. A month before his death, the dentist urged his patients to be tested for the HIV. Four more of his patients tested positive for the virus, and further testing established a close relationship.

This brings us to another issue: do health practitioners need to be tested for HIV, and if yes, should the results be made public? This is definitely a crux of a thorny debate. From a patient's standpoint it would be a resounding yes. However, the issue is much more complex. If the new measures were to require the testing of doctors and health workers for the AIDS virus, they could violate many state laws that require informed consent and that protect confidentiality of test results. Add to this the personal cost of losing professional livelihood and discrimination, and the issue becomes more blurred.

I think it makes sense to test health practitioners who are involved in performing invasive procedures on patients. The CDC should establish strict guidelines on how to deal with a doctor who tests positive, to protect both the patient and doctor as much as possible.

If a court ruling handed down in New Jersey in April of 1991 is any indication, mandatory disclosure is the wave of the future. This state went even further. Because of growing anxiety among healthcare workers, the medical society of New Jersey called for mandatory testing of all hospital patients. However, if this is carried out, there is a danger of discrimination against people with the virus, leading to possible segregation and loss of health insurance and adequate medical treatment. The CDC, the general public and the medical profession won't stop debating these issues any time soon. It's possible that the courts will be the final arbiters in this debate.

   * Artificial insemination

With more couples opting for artificial insemination to conceive children, another (although infrequent) invasion path for the AIDS virus is possible. Screening tests for AIDS, in addition to an investigative history of sexual partners of semen donors, are currently being used by many artificial insemination centers. Women contemplating artificial insemination should ask about each center's policy to reduce likelihood of the spread of AIDS.

   * AIDS and mosquito bites: scare or reality?

The mosquito is the most common carrier of arboviruses, which are a family of viruses that can also be transmitted by fleas and ticks. While scientists so far have not been able to confirm mechanical transmission by mosquitoes, some recent disturbing findings have raised new concerns. One of these findings is the transmission by mosquitoes of HTLV-1, a human retrovirus related to HIV (the AIDS virus) and associated with T-cell leukemia. Another study, done at a private laboratory in Rockville, Md., showed that two days after feeding mosquitoes with AIDS-tainted blood, the virus was still found in the stomach of some of the insects.

Attention to this route of possible transmission was first drawn through the case of Belle Glade, a Florida farming community. This community has the highest rate of AIDS per capita — 375 per 100,000. What is important about these cases is that half of them occur among non-risk groups, so other factors must be involved. It has been suggested that the dampness (see Chapter Two) and exposure to mosquitoes, and other unknown organisms, could encourage infection with the AIDS virus. Remember also that candida albicans, or yeast, thrives in warm, moist climates; chronic yeast infections could substantially weaken the immune systems of these people.

The good news about the mosquito scare is that various labs show that the AIDS virus fails to reproduce and multiply inside the mosquito. However, I think that we forget to take into consideration the many factors involved in the weakening of the immune system, especially climatic factors, emotions and the concomitant presence of other viruses and yeast cells.

* AIDS and Organ Transplants: A Forgotten Way of Transmission

Painfully illustrative of the lapse of time that occurs between HIV infection and positivity of the HIV ELISA test, is the case of a man who was shot to death in October, 1985 and whose tissue samples were given to 52 patients. Although the deceased person was tested negative for AIDS, three of the tissue recipients have tested positive for the virus and three have died of AIDS as of May 15, 1991. The three patients that died received the infected donor's heart and kidneys. It is obvious that this tragic case will be the object of a careful study by the FDA to prevent future cases and maximize the safety of organ and tissue transplants. One possibility would be the use of the PCR test mentioned in this chapter.

Possible Co-Factors in Contracting AIDS

The viruses and disease-causing agents discussed below do not lead to AIDS directly. But when an immune system has been weakened by battling one of these conditions, it may become more susceptible to invasion by the AIDS virus. A short discussion of each follows.

HTLV-1, AIDS' *Cancer-Causing Cousin*

HTLV-1 is the first virus ever shown to cause cancer in humans — a rare and fatal form of leukemia or, less often, a neurological disorder resembling multiple sclerosis.

A study of drug users in New Orleans and New Jersey, run by the National Cancer Institute, found that almost half of them were carriers of the HTLV-1 virus. This virus targets the same immune system cells as the AIDS virus: the T-lymphocytes, the directors of the immune system. The origin of this virus remains a mystery. Dr. Robert Gallo, one of the co-discoverers of the virus, thinks it originates in Africa, while Japanese scientists traced it back to thousand of years ago when Japan was settled by central Asians.

There is good and bad news with this virus. The good news is it seems to be less virulent than the AIDS virus, and requires more than a single exposure to cause disease. The bad news is that we don't know how long it can remain dormant before it causes leukemia. And it spreads by the same route as the AIDS virus: from sexual or other direct contact with blood and body fluids. To be on the safe side, until more data is gathered, tests for HTLV-1 are done by the American Red Cross for large-scale screening of this cancerous cousin of AIDS.

Herpes Simplex *Viruses and Candida*

As we discussed in the chapter introduction, the herpes simplex viruses and candida albicans cause immune-suppressed conditions. People with herpes simplex viruses or candida will be more susceptible to AIDS upon contact with a carrier's blood or semen. The absence of such "co-factors" explains why some individuals, in spite of close contact with an AIDS victim, do not show antibodies against the virus: their immune systems are not chronically weaken-ed by other viruses or yeast cells.

In the case of retroviruses, a new virus called HBLV — for Human B-Cell Lymphotrophic Virus — was isolated in Dr. Robert Gallo's lab. Although Gallo is not ready to say this virus is connected with any illness, I am convinced that it is another epiphenomena in the CFIDS outbreaks throughout the United States. HBLV is thought to be yet another member of the herpes family, but there is no evidence at this point that HBLV is sexually transmitted. To date, most of the AIDS patients have not been found positive for HBLV; it has only been isolated from those with B-cell lymphomas.

If doctors tested their AIDS patients for herpes simplex viruses and candida, I suspect they would find a high incidence of both conditions, higher than in the normal population. In fact, I have no doubt that almost 100% of the AIDS patients have at the same time CMV, EBV, candida, herpes simplex I and II, HHV-6, hepatitis B virus and also Entamoeba Histolytica or Giardiasis. A study done by Loffler, et al., in 1986, showed the presence of Candidiasis in autopsies of AIDS patients in the mouth, esophagus and large intestine, as well as candida abscesses in the liver. This information becomes frightening when we see that most young candida patients simultaneously have EBV, CMV and possible parasites in their body. In my view, they are more susceptible to all other infections, AIDS included, if they don't get proper care. Which condition comes first, we don't know. But there is the sense of a unique relationship between the group of immuno-suppressed diseases (herpes simplex group, syphilis and candida) and the AIDS outbreak.

Symptoms and Stages of the Disease

Many candidiasis and CFIDS patients fear that they have at least ARC (AIDS-related complex) or AIDS before their diagnosis is made correctly. Some doctors contribute to this confusion, and in view of the similarity of the symptoms of the above conditions, it is almost understandable. However, AIDS phenomena are classically divided into four groups, according to their severity:

Asymptomatic HIV-*positive* AIDS *patients*

At this stage of exposure, there are no clinical signs, and there is no laboratory abnormality in the ratio of T_4 to T_8 white blood cells.

LAS, *or* AIDS *patients with Lymphadenopathy Syndrome*

These patients show characteristic swelling of at least two or more lymphatic nodes, apart from those in the groin area, for longer than three months.

ARC, *or* AIDS-*related complex*

Patients show at least two of the following symptoms for more than three months: decrease in physical and mental powers, night sweats, increased transpiration, loss of weight (greater than 10% of total body weight), fever of unknown origin, diarrhea, fungi,

Herpes Simplex, Herpes Zoster and impaired wound-healing. In this stage, we frequently see an increase in T8 or T-suppressor cells.

Full-blown AIDS

This condition includes persistent and recurrent opportunistic infections, indicating defects of the immune system, as well as malignant tumors such as Kaposi's sarcoma. There are several target organs involved:
* The skin reveals herpes simplex blisters in the oral, anal and genital mucosae; the Kaposi's sarcoma produces nodes of red and black color in skin, mucosae, spleen, liver and brain.
* The gastrointestinal tract shows candida infections being the cause of prolonged diarrhea (lasting longer than one month).
* The lungs are often infected by pneumocystis Carinii (in approximately 60% of all AIDS patients). Other infections with Toxoplasma, candida, Cryptococcus, CMV, EBV and tuberculosis have been widely recognized.
* Central nervous system involvement: It is now clear that 30% to 60% of AIDS patients develop a syndrome of dementia characterized by memory loss, inability to concentrate and lethargy. No one knows exactly how widespread this AIDS-related dementia is, but autopsies show that 80% of AIDS patients have at least some central nervous system disease.

The mental decline in AIDS-related dementia can be gradual or precipitous, and it can strike early or late in the course of the disease. Ten percent of AIDS patients develop dementia as a first symptom. This was slowly recognized by doctors, since AIDS dementia can masquerade as classical mental illness, simulating anxiety attacks, depression and also hallucinations. The virus' presence in the brain also vastly complicates efforts to develop an effective treatment for the disease. Any drug for AIDS would have to pass the blood-brain barrier that allows only vital components to get into the brain. AZT is the first and only drug so far that can handle this first hurdle. But whether AZT is effective once it gets into the brain is unclear.

Diagnosis: Testing and Its Dilemmas

Many doctors now feel that testing and early diagnosis and treatment can forestall development of full-blown AIDS. However, many do not want to be tested, believing that a result of HIV-positive would have negative effects on their lives. But by avoiding the issue, one raises two questions with perhaps incompatible answers, one of ethics and one of emotional well-being.

Do high-risk individuals have an ethical obligation to be tested, for the sake of past and future sexual partners?

Does the lack of a cure make the test irrelevant as long as safe sex is practiced? Fear, of course, is the main reason why most people avoid the testing. If more treatment drugs were developed, one would see a lot more people coming in for testing. People ask themselves: "What is the advantage of the test, and can I deal with the results?"

Another hazard is the existent confidentiality law. Currently, it is illegal for doctors to inform anyone but the patient of test results. Under these laws, doctors cannot tell wives when their husbands test positive; neither can they tell nurses that they are treating somebody with AIDS. It is clear that endangered third parties should have the right to protect themselves.

Questions about who should be tested, how testing can be kept confidential — or if it should be — and the medical, legal and ethical consequences of testing are piling up, with no ready answers in sight. While the debate continues, millions of already infected Americans are passing it on to many millions more. Of course, the best way to prevent this is to find those carriers, and warn them about changing their sex habits, and hope they will comply with this precaution. It is clear that testing has to start somewhere; but since it is impossible and too expensive to test everyone, who should be tested?

The government might consider mandatory testing for exposure to the AIDS virus for pregnant women, couples applying for marriage licenses, people seeking treatment for other sexually transmitted diseases, and all patients admitted to hospitals. The federal government now requires AIDS testing for active-duty military personnel, recruits and Foreign Service officers. All donated blood is also screened. Would this resolve all our problems? No. For one thing, even this massive screening would fail to identify recently infected patients, since it can take to up to a year before antibodies show up in the blood.

The Available Tests

The primary test is the ELISA (short for Enzyme-Linked Immuno- Sorbent Assay) test. About 5cc of blood is drawn, and the blood is screened for any antibodies that have been produced in response to the AIDS virus. Running the test takes about three hours. If the result of the ELISA is negative, testing stops, since there are almost no false negatives. Among the people most likely to have AIDS, false negatives may occur if the test is given within six months after infection.

Two positive ELISAs are the signal for a more precise test — the Western Blot. In the Western Blot, viral proteins are blotted onto special paper. A specific pattern will appear on the paper if AIDS antibodies are present. After two positive ELISAs, a positive Western Blot means that the person probably is infected. But even then, the tests should be repeated in three to six months.

* Margins of Error

However, a study done by the federal government's Office of Technology Assessment found that tests can be very inaccurate indeed. For groups at low risk, which will be the majority of people deliberately taking a test, 90% of the positive findings are so-called *"false positives,"* indicating infection where none exists. So nine out of ten hear this dreadful news — positive for AIDS — when, in fact, the virus is not at all present. Imagine the consequences!

For high-risk people, on the other hand, we have the opposite: the test produces false *negatives* about 10% of the time, meaning that 1 in 10 of these people are told they are not infected when in fact they are. These margins of error have devastating emotional and public-health consequences. They provide an argument against mass screening.

* Dealing with Time Lag

A new study on gay men in Finland also found that some who became infected with the AIDS virus did not form antibodies for *more than one year.* This is far longer than most experts had expected. The study was done at the University of Tampere in Finland by Dr. Kai Krohn. The new finding means that some people may have been declared free of the virus prematurely, before antibodies appeared in their blood.

The big drawback with the ELISA test is the time-lag problem: as mentioned before, it can take up to six months before an infected person has formed antibodies against the HIV. In other words, people who are actually infected may be told that they are negative, allowing further spreading of the virus.

There is some good news on the horizon: a new test, called Polymerase Chain Reaction (PCR), will overcome this major flaw.

PCR testing detects HIV within days or hours after infection. Two California labs have been licensed by the state to perform the PCR test:

Specialty Laboratories Inc.
2211 Michigan Avenue
Santa Monica, California 90404
phone: (213) 828-6543

Pathology Institute
2920 Telegraph Avenue
Berkeley, California 94705
phone: (415) 540-1638

There are two groups who might be wise to ask for this test: pregnant women who are worried that they might have been exposed to HIV, since the fetus can become infected with the HIV before the ELISA test will detect a recent infection; and people who tested negative with the ELISA, but whose lifestyles — unsafe sex or intravenous drug use, puts them at high risk.

Other Important Lab Features of HIV *Infection*

Most patients with HIV infection eventually develop profound T-cell deficiency. Immunological features of AIDS are expressed below:

* Marked decrease of T_4 cells
* Normal or increased T_8 cells
* Abnormal B cell (antibody) function
* Impaired natural killer cell activity
* Decreased interferon and interleukin-2 production
* Decreased T_4/T_8 ratio
* Decreased lymphocyte count
* Negative delayed hypersensitivity skin tests

Comparing this laboratory profile with the CFIDS profile in Chapter Four, you can clearly see the similarities.

It is clear from the above that there is no strict rule available about testing yet. What will happen in the future is uncertain.

Therapy for AIDS and HIV-Positive Patients

With no apparent cure for AIDS in sight, AIDS sufferers are easy prey for hundreds of quack remedies or doctors peddling half-truths and false hopes. This section of the chapter will present the available therapies to these patients. As with all other immune-suppressed patients, HIV-positive and AIDS sufferers should follow as healthful a lifestyle as possible. Therefore, Section Three of this book should be read and followed with special interest by these individuals.

The FDA is looking for ways to improve its notoriously bureaucratic drug-approval process. Because this disease is so devastating, the FDA has eased up its stringent rules, and is making some drugs available for those with no alternative therapies in sight.

The major hope, of course, is that a vaccine will soon be developed. In this section, we will also discuss the search for a viable vaccine. And finally, a review of safe sex practices to help prevent infection in the first place.

Search for a Vaccine

Dr. Daniel Zagury, a French researcher at the Pierre and Marie Curie University, was the first researcher to test an AIDS vaccine on human volunteers in Zaire, Africa. Dr. Zagury disclosed that he himself was the first one to receive this vaccination. "I considered this to be the only ethical line of conduct," he told reporters. So far, Dr. Zagury has suffered no side-effects from the vaccination. Within 30 days of taking the vaccine, laboratory studies showed that his blood serum was "highly positive" for antibodies against one major strain of the AIDS virus. However, none of the volunteers was deliberately exposed to AIDS to test the vaccine. This experimental vaccine was designed to stimulate a second kind of immune system defense, called cell-medicated response, in which special blood cells also fight invading microorganisms.

Following a series of four self-injections that began in November, 1986, and continued through 1987, Dr. Zagury has suffered no ill effects. He has developed what appears to be the strongest human immunity yet achieved against the virus. It clearly indicates that he achieved the expected immunity from the vaccine, which is hopeful if one compares this to previous experience with other vaccinations. The only thing that has not been shown is whether it protects against the AIDS virus.

As American volunteers are being asked to sign up for the first experimental vaccine, scientists are wrestling with complex technical and ethical questions as to how to conduct such studies and protect the volunteers. Investigators will have to enlist thousands of suitable subjects, monitor them for years, and somehow prove that the vaccine is effective without exposing them to AIDS. To get volunteers for this study will be difficult at best. But is this so surprising? These vaccinated volunteers become HIV-positive, a considerable health concern as well as a social stigma for anybody in the future. Will these volunteers be protected against discrimination in jobs, housing and medical treatment? Will they risk losing their health insurance, leaving them unprotected for any disease or injury?

In 1987 a small Connecticut firm, MicroGeneSys, Inc., became the first to win approval from the FDA to use their vaccine on human beings. Scientists have no evidence that the prototype, known as Vax-Syn, prevents infection by the AIDS virus in humans. But animals that received inoculations reacted as the vaccine makers had hoped: they developed antibodies, that—theoretically, at least — can render the virus harmless. But much remains to be done. Tests must be conducted to establish whether the vaccine has any harmful side-effects, and whether it really works. Even the most optimistic sources do not expect any vaccine ready for mass injection for another five years. Each stage of testing presents formidable hurdles.

* AIDS Antibodies Mysterious

First there is the mystery of AIDS antibodies. Most vaccines work by forming antibodies capable of defending our system against many disease-causing organisms. However, it is not yet known if an AIDS vaccination will follow the same pattern. Most AIDS sufferers do have antibodies to the virus. However, this apparently does not provide them with protection, given the progressive course of the disease. In other words, simply because a vaccine spurs production of AIDS antibodies does not necessarily mean that it will fend off the virus.

* Virus Mutates

Most viruses, and especially the AIDS virus, undergo mutation, which means that an inoculation against one variety could be useless against another one.

* Concern About Side Effects

The good news about developing an AIDS vaccine is that widely different strains of the deadly virus share common "soft spots" that can be attacked by antibodies. It suggests that scientists may not have far to go. However, some experts fear that in the long run the presence of AIDS antibodies may disrupt the immune systems of individuals who get the vaccine.

Vaccines against AIDS raise many additional questions about safety and effectiveness. A vaccine, of course, will not help those already suffering from the disease. So the immediate hope is that medications can be used to ease suffering and prolong life.

Medications

While no cure has been found for AIDS, progress is being made in developing antiviral, immune-modulating agents to treat the disease. The FDA has given top priority to all potential AIDS drugs.

* Retrovir (AZT)

More commonly known as AZT, Retrovir was the first approved drug for AIDS. The FDA's approval of this drug took less than four months, quite a record when the normal process takes several years and millions of dollars in research. The drug was tested in a classic double-blind study, where 50% of the patients received the drug and the other 50% received a placebo. Since the results were extremely favorable, with fewer deaths in the AZT group than the placebo group, it was concluded that it would be unethical not to make the drug available to treat all patients. There was also less incidence of opportunistic infections and an initial increase in the T4 cells in the AZT group.

Unfortunately, as with most medications, there are side-effects. In particular, anemia occurred in about 40%, necessitating multiple transfusions. The toxicity of the drug and our limited experience with it dampen enthusiasm for its use. Better news was that half of the initial advised dosage of AZT was still effective, cutting down on its disadvantages. However, it is also important to remember that the long-term effects of AZT are unknown and that AZT therapy has not been shown to reduce the risk of transmission of HIV to others.

Several potential AIDS therapies are being clinically researched but are not yet approved by the FDA. Under the Freedom of Information Act, FDA employees are prohibited from publicly discussing the status of drugs under the agency's review. However, many of the sponsors of experimental drugs have made some information available. Isoprinosine, Thymopentin, Riboviran, Ampligen, Alpha Interferon, Dextran Sulfate and Interleukin-2 are just a few of those products.

Another problem researchers are attempting to deal with is the increasing danger of children contracting AIDS, when borne by mothers infected with the AIDS virus. Because the nervous systems of children are still developing, these young victims are even more vulnerable to AIDS-related neurological disorders. No therapeutic agents are currently available to prevent infection in newborns. Researchers at Harvard Medical School developed a surrogate model with pregnant mice and tested the effectiveness of AZT. While AZT did not prevent infection, newborn mice lived longer and had a dramatic increase in survival. Also encouraging was the fact that the mice were born without any deformities. It is clear that a similar model will be used to test future anti-viral drugs.

* Therapies to "Confuse" the Virus

Attacking the AIDS virus directly with medications is just one tactic used by scientists. Another approach is to confuse this deadly virus with ingenious tactics. As already noted, the AIDS virus penetrates an immune cell (T4) by clinging to a protein receptor (called CD4). Once it attaches to this receptor, it has in effect opened a secret passageway past the "General" of the immune system, and the battle is usually lost.

Scientists have come up with a cunning device; they have made copies of this CD4 receptor, and added them to test tubes containing both healthy cells and the HIV. The "imposter" receptors neutralize these AIDS viruses through a mechanism known as competitive inhibition. In lay-person's terms, that means that if we put more CD4 receptors in our blood, the HIV will make no distinction between these "false" receptors and the real receptors, and therefore will bind to any of them and neutralize them. A drawback at this time is that we do not know if this form of therapy will help people already infected, with or without symptoms. Yet it is an interesting approach, currently being investigated and researched by various companies. (See Figure #8)

* Treating Secondary Infections

While extensive studies are being done for medications that kill the virus, other scientists focus on developing medications to combat the exotic and deadly infections that AIDS victims contract. Pneumocystis Carinii pneumonia, a lung disorder, is a common complication of AIDS. It is caused by protozoa, one celled-organisms. Similar to yeast cells, these protozoa exist in the body and are kept in check by the immune system, but go haywire when the system is

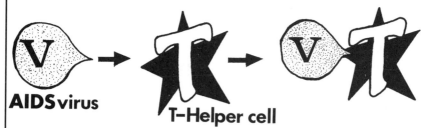

AIDSvirus   T-Helper cell

The AIDS virus invades the T-Helper cell by clinging to a protein receptor.

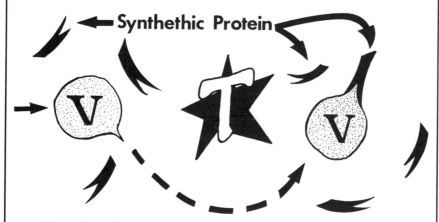

Synthethic Protein

CD4 binds to the AIDS virus and through competitive inhibition, arrests the invasion.

fig 8

In the upper drawing, we see how the AIDS virus invades the T-Helper cell. In the lower drawing, the AIDS virus is "tricked" into avoiding the T-Helper cell by a synthetic protein called CD4.

suppressed, caused by some treatments such as cancer chemo-therapy or by immune-suppressing conditions such as AIDS.

In a new approach by doctors at the National Institutes of Health and George Washington University Medical Center, a combination of two drugs is used: an anticancer drug, trimetrexate, together with leucovorin, a protective agent against the toxic effects of the first drug. Many of the patients in the study actually recover from this pneumonia. Until studies are conducted on a larger scale, it is still too early to assess the efficacy of this new therapeutic approach. Bactrim, a well-known broad spectrum antibiotic, is often administered to fight this pneumonia.

Working on Prevention

It is clear that the fight against AIDS must take place on multiple fronts: in the research labs where vaccines and effective medications are being developed, in the legislatures where monies are allocated for research and guidelines for ethical protection are passed, and in public health education, where professionals work to prevent further infection with this virus.

* Condoms

A disease such as AIDS is a "marketing dream" for condom manufacturers. With the support of former Surgeon General C. Everett Koop and even the Catholic Church, condoms are "in." However, simply using a condom does not automatically ensure protection. Recent studies have indicated that natural membrane condoms are not able to protect against the HIV virus. For once, "close to nature" is not the best solution. Therefore, FDA allows only latex condoms to be labeled as suitable for the prevention of sexually transmitted diseases, including AIDS.

To maximize protection against these diseases, it is important that condoms be used properly. Following are some important and simple rules (it is amazing how little is known about them by the public):

- Use a condom every time you have sexual intercourse.
- When you buy it, the condom is rolled up in a small package. Put the condom on over the tip of the penis as soon as it is hard, and before you and your partner get close.

- Unroll the condom onto the penis until the entire penis is covered. After ejaculation, pull the penis out immediately (hold onto the condom to make sure it comes out too!).
- Remove the condom, do not use again!

It is not a bad idea to use a spermicide with the condom — a contraceptive foam, jelly or cream. Since there can be leakage of the condom, and natural condoms made of lamb intestines contain microscopic pores large enough to allow invasion of the HIV, additional protective measures are not a luxury. Condoms fail to prevent pregnancy about 10% of the time, so that statistic must make us wary of the transmission danger of AIDS.

Alternative Therapies

Because of the lack of apparent success with any of the existing drugs, patients increasingly look for other ways to improve their health. Even doctors, until now mostly intolerant of any alternative approach, appear increasingly receptive to the idea. In this area common sense is the best guide. A genuine and humane approach would start with candor: "I don't want to tell you that it does not help, because I simply don't know!"

The next section of this book, on therapeutic techniques, contains many of these alternative, noninvasive (nondamaging) approaches. These include following a healthy eating program, taking immunity-boosting supplements and making important lifestyle changes. After all, only the strength of your immune system is capable of guaranteeing you full protection from these diseases. AIDS is not just a disease of the immune system. It is a disease of courage and hope in the face of death. To all victims I would like to say: turn this into a challenge, a challenge to live a long, healthy, productive life. Let HIV become a more positive influence in your life than a negative one. Become a more focused, settled person. Have good, loving relationships, and cherish a supportive family and friends. You are not powerless, you can do a lot more than just wait. This goes for the family and friends as well, to whom I have written an "open letter," presented in Chapter Fourteen at the end of this book. I hope that it will be a helpful tool to stimulate communication between friends and family alike.

SECTION THREE

A NEW UNDERSTANDING OF HEALTH AND IMMUNITY

CHAPTER NINE

THERAPIES FOR VIRAL AND YEAST INFECTIONS

Chapters Four through Eight described the major illnesses and their symptoms. Once your condition has been correctly diagnosed, what do you do? In this chapter, we'll talk about the various therapies, mainstream and alternative, that have been found useful in treating patients with viral illness, candidiasis and CFIDS. As you recall, Chapter Seven gave the therapies for parasites and Chapter Eight the therapies for AIDS.

Therapy for Viral Illness

"Go home, rest, and hope that it will pass soon," is the advice patients frequently hear when they consult their doctors about a viral illness. This may suffice for someone with a mild case of the flu. But to a person with CFIDS, it's not very encouraging. The condition is not only debilitating, it's baffling: patients go from feeling perfectly healthy, to suddenly incapacitated, a fraction of their former selves.

Nevertheless, this section does include current mainstream treatments, such as rest, prescribed for other viral illnesses. The treatments are presented with their pros and cons. For additional methods, however, you should also turn to Chapter Twelve. That will give you ways to actually get better and to boost a suppressed immune system. Since some of the following treatments have helped some patients, they are worth mentioning.

Can You Really Rest Easy?

Do you feel too tired to put one foot in front of the other? It seems a logical step that rest is the best advice we can give you. Never has this advice been given so frequently to a specific class of patients. I think this is wrong to some degree. Don't misunderstand me. I know people with viral illnesses are tired; but think for a moment. Have you ever sat on your sofa all day watching TV or stayed in bed, doing nothing? How will you feel at the end of such a day? Even if you are completely healthy, you will feel very tired!

It is simple: inactivity can lead to stagnation, including stagnation of your energy. If not used, nothing will work properly anymore. If you don't keep active to some degree, your organs will start functioning at 50% of their strength, creating a real "back-up" of toxins, causing more symptoms. Thus, you create a vicious circle of lassitude and of heaviness.

But do not misinterpret the message of "some activity." If you are a CFIDS patients, you should not be preparing for the next Olympic Games. With viral involvement, complete rest is sometimes the only solution for the initial period of infection.

* Activities to Try:

If you are actively doing something to improve your condition, you should try *certain* exercises. The best one to try first is walking. You can do it alone or with a friend for emotional support, and at the pace you want. As I said, even this is impossible for some CFIDS patients and they should not force the issue. If you feel more tired after the exercise and need several days to recuperate, you should lay off for at least another week. But you should try again! But remember. At least half of all CFIDS victims *can* walk right away and should do so. Other excellent exercises are stretching, yoga and bicycling. It is interesting to see that even when patients feel they cannot move their limbs, the majority feel better after the exercise. Any exercise involving a lot of muscle bulk should be avoided, especially weight lifting, tennis, running or strenuous aerobics.

* When to Exercise:

The best time to do your exercise is right at the beginning of the day, even before breakfast. By getting rid of toxins accumulated during the night, you will benefit the whole day! Before starting the exercise, drink an 8-oz. glass of warm water with lemon juice; the cleansing will be more complete.

Will Medications Do the Trick?

Sinequan

This drug is a tricyclic antidepressant with potent antihistaminic and anti-inflammatory effects. Usually the dosage is at least 40 mg (per day). The dosage used for these CFIDS or virally ill patients is usually 10 mg taken at night. A few patients find relief with this method. Sinequan is prescribed in doses far below those recom-mended for the treatment of depression. According to advocates of this medication, these small doses could stimulate or modulate the immune system.

Sometimes, when 10 mg does not work, the dose is increased, but usually not to more than 30 mg. As a drug therapy, I probably would advise patients to take this one first. Sinequan is used in big medical centers by infectious disease doctors as a sole treatment in CFIDS patients. Personally, I have discovered that it only seems to help in about 10% of the cases and only for a short time. The most positive reaction I have seen is the diminishment of insomnia, a constant symptom of CFIDS. If no positive reaction is noticed after two months of the medication, it's probably advisable to discontinue it.

Tagamet ™ *(Cimetidine)*

This is the top selling medication in many countries, but not for treating CFIDS. It is a potent medication prescribed mostly for stomach disorder, especially ulcers. How was this introduced in treating CFIDS? Researchers observed that very young children, who have no suppressor T-cells, (because of their immature immune systems), often have no symptoms when they have an EBV infection. Suppressor T-cells have receptors for Cimetidine, which would decrease their function. By taking this drug, some patients showed some improvement. However, the symptoms seemed to come back after the therapy was stopped. A similar pattern was found with Zantac ™, another medication for stomach disorders, which also had to be taken indefinitely.

Acyclovir (Zovirax ™*)*

Acyclovir was the first antiviral drug approved for use in the U.S., in 1985. It was chiefly used in the battle against herpes simplex II or genital herpes. Since EBV, CMV and HHV-6 belong to the family of herpes simplex viruses, some researchers tried to use it for CFIDS. However, the drug seems to have very little effect on any virus but H. simplex I and II. It is an expensive drug, and in my opinion, it is a waste of time and money to use it for CFIDS except for suppressing the recurrent flare-ups of genital herpes, common in CFIDS patients.

Injections

Holistic and nutritionally oriented doctors have found various injections, including vitamin solutions, to be beneficial. The first indicated is vitamin C, and there is no doubt that vitamin C, given in an intravenous push or drip, will benefit the patient greatly. Linus Pauling, the father of vitamin C therapy, advises doses orally up to 30,000 mg if tolerated (loose stools indicate you should cut back).

* Often, vitamin C, given intravenously in dosages of 10,000 to 20,000 milligrams at a time, delivers an instant energy boost to CFIDS patients, providing the much-needed ray of hope. Usually the vitamin C is mixed with calcium, magnesium and B complex vitamins in a ratio of 1 cc of each to 15 cc vitamin C. Be aware of any possible corn allergies, since most vitamin C intravenous preparations are derived from corn. Patients allergic to corn should avoid this way of administering vitamin C. In certain parts of the country, vitamin C derived from rose hips is available; this would be an acceptable alternative.

* Another proven energy stimulus with these patients are injections with desiccated liver, folic acid, AMP and pantothenic acid (B_5). Two injections a week for several weeks will help CFIDS sufferers.

* Injections with Kutapressin ™, a mixture of polypeptides derived from porcine liver, have been given for decades in holistic practices and proven, in the same way as the above injections, to be helpful. At the moment, Kutapressin ™ seems to be one of the favored therapies for CFIDS given by mainstream doctors. Daily injections for up to 10 days, followed by three injections a week until recovery, are recommended. Until more is known about the exact mechanism of Kutapressin ™, you should not expect wonders from this therapy. Talk to a holistic doctor who has experience with this method, and ask his or her opinion of its effectiveness.

Although some provide modest improvement, the above therapies are not the solution. The good news is that more long-lasting help is available, through:

1) a specific diet (discussed in Chapter Eleven)
2) a newly discovered therapy with herbal products (discussed in Chapter Ten) and
3) new ways to boost and support your immune system (discussed in Chapter Thirteen).

Therapy for Candidiasis

Head Off Yeast Overgrowth

The first and best treatment of any disease is the prevention of it. It's important that you pay close attention to all the triggering factors (from the questionnaire in Chapter One and as described in Chapter Two).

* Avoid Triggering Factors

You should be especially alert to the triggering factor of antibiotic overuse. Antibiotics are quite effective in knocking out bacterial infection, but they have no effect on viral conditions. Nevertheless, physicians sometimes prescribe them anyway, often when patients beg for some medicine to make them better. The problem is that antibiotics, besides attacking the "bad" bacteria, also kill off the "good" bacteria that your intestines need to function properly. With no bacteria present, that leaves a vacuum in which candida albicans can flourish. So, use of antibiotics can be a triggering factor in causing candidiasis.

Of course, there are many indications for antibiotic intake. There are ways to protect yourself from adverse effects when you take the medication.

* Take a high daily dose of acidophilus (2 TBS of liquid). This will go a long way toward eliminating the side effect of diarrhea that accompanies antibiotic intake. If you have been told that yogurt will accomplish the same thing as acidophilus, this is not true. There is a negligible concentration of friendly bacteria; you need a higher amount to counteract the antibiotics.

* Patients who are on any antifungal medication should double their dosage for the duration of the antibiotic intake. Even for those patients who have not taken any medication, a maintenance dosage of an antifungal medication is advised.

Battle Plan for Candidiasis

By taking acidophilus, you'll be doing your part to counteract the triggering properties of antibiotics. Once you have candidiasis, as established by the diagnostic criteria in Chapter Six, you will need to combat it. Here are the objectives:

* Starve the Candida
* Kill the Candida
* Replace the Normal Flora
* Starve the Yeast, or the Anti-Yeast Diet

Most of us "live to eat" instead of eating to live. Unfortunately, much of our social life centers around food intake, which does not make it easier for a person to choose not to eat the regular diet. But eating properly for your particular needs simply makes good sense.

As we will discuss in the chapter on eating for peak immunity, there are many reasons for eating besides hunger. Adults often use sweets as a way to reward or comfort children. Often, as adults, we use food as a way to fill an emotional void. We sit down to eat and do not want to stop. The purpose of "shoving the food in" is to fill that bottomless emotional hole which, of course, can never be filled by eating. Often, it is only by trying to change your diet that you become aware of these counterproductive lifetime habits.

Keeping in mind that candida cells are voracious eaters, consuming almost anything for their growth, you need to pay attention to their favorite foods: *carbohydrates* (especially sugars) and *fermented* foods. (See the Appendix for "Autobiography of a Yeast Cell.")

The basic tenet of this phase of the battle plan, "starve the candida," therefore, revolves around eliminating processed carbohydrates, sugars and fermented foods. The eating plan that encompasses this is described in Chapter Eleven. That diet is not only for sufferers of candidiasis. In reality, it's a peak immunity diet.

* Kill the Candida

After suffering from over-medication, most patients are not very enthusiastic about returning to any medication. This is understandable. However, candidiasis is a serious condition. It will require an anti-yeast medication to break the cycle of yeast cell overgrowth which is debilitating to your immune system. So, after starving an enemy by blocking the food supply lines, you also need to attack the fortress to ensure his defeat.

Choosing the best weapon is the most important step. There are two types: natural products and medications.

1. NATURAL PRODUCTS

* Garlic

Garlic has a long history of medicinal use. It dates back to the Babylonians, the Pharaohs and the Greeks. Louis Pasteur, the famous microbiologist, and more recently, Albert Schweitzer, were firm believers in garlic for its antimicrobial and antibacterial activity. Garlic is a natural antifungal agent, and can be helpful for candidiasis patients. It is often the *only* thing that can relieve bloating and gas. It lessens the intestinal pain and burning that are often experienced by candidiasis sufferers. Fresh garlic in salads also relieves water retention in the body.

If you can't take digestive enzymes, garlic will help you to digest food. Take at least two tablespoons of liquid garlic mixed in either water or juice, or at least six deodorized capsules with each meal.

There's another plus when you take garlic regularly: it's been shown to effectively lower cholesterol levels in the blood.

* Pau d'Arco

This is a South American herb which is often referred to by its other Spanish names: Ipe Roxa, Lapacho and Taheebo. It is currently hailed for its effects in curing abdominal cancer (in South America) and candidiasis.

Pau d'Arco is the inner bark of a large tree that flowers in a vibrant pink, purple or yellow, depending on the species. Throughout South America Pau d'Arco is used as a remedy for immune system-related problems, such as colds, fevers, infections and snake bites, but even more important for us, the bark has natural anti-fungal properties. It was one of the major healing herbs used by the Incas. The toxicity of Pau d'Arco is very low. It may loosen the bowels, but that is frequently desirable for a patient with candidiasis. It is available in capsules, tinctures, tea bags, and bulk form. Usual dosage is up to two cups of tea a day or two capsules daily. Some people may be sensitive or allergic to Pau d'Arco, so start this program under the supervision of your doctor. It also acts as a diuretic, important to remember when losing too many fluids with gastrointestinal disorders.

2. ANTIFUNGAL DRUGS AND SUPPLEMENTS

* Nystatin Powder

Nystatin powder was the initial drug of choice in treating candidiasis. However, at this point it is totally outdated — and for very good reasons. First of all, it is rather expensive and very few pharmacies carry it. A major disadvantage is that Nystatin is *not* a broad-spectrum fungicide. While effective for certain strains of candida, many pathogenic fungi are unaffected by it. With prolonged use, it leads to the development of resistance to the drug and continued symptoms. Nystatin is a mold by-product and may cause allergic reactions in the mold-sensitive patient.

Some adverse reactions are nausea and vomiting. Patients may experience withdrawal symptoms when the Nystatin is discontinued. In the generic sense, Nystatin is a potent antibiotic and the long-term effects of its use on normal bacterial and normal fungal intestinal flora are not clear.

Because of these serious side effects, it might be wise to question your physician if he or she prescribes Nystatin as the only therapy for systemic candidiasis. A trial of Nystatin therapy for candida overgrowth was published in *The New England Journal of Medicine* on December 20, 1990. The researchers concluded that "Nystatin does not reduce systemic or psychological symptoms significantly more than placebo in women with presumed candidiasis hypersensitivity syndrome." [1] This study merely confirms what holistic doctors have known for years. Even more validity could be given to its conclusions if some of the more recent medications, such as Nizarol or Diflucan, were also studied. Also, to have any success in combatting yeast, no matter what the medication will be, a diet change should have been proposed to the patients in this study.

Despite these cautionary notes, Nystatin can be used locally for vaginal discharge and itching, or it can be sniffed to alleviate postnasal drip. And it is most effective when prescribed to counteract the frequent painful urination the patient experiences at night and during the day. For this symptom, you can start with 1/8th of a tsp building it up to 1/2 tsp twice a day.

For this medication, you need to obtain a prescription from your doctor. Be sure that the pharmacist does not give you the *topical* powder. You need the *oral* powder. This can be taken for several weeks without any problem under the supervision of your doctor, who will determine the precise doses you should take.

* Nizarol tablets, 200 mg (Ketoconazole)

This is a very potent antifungal drug. It is a synthetic broad-spectrum antifungal agent available in white tablets, each containing 200 mg ketoconazole.

In my opinion, it is not a first-line drug for systemic candidiasis since adverse reactions such as nausea and vomiting and, more disturbing, liver damage, can occur. A blood test before and after use of it is mandatory. It is easy to take, since only one tablet daily is required.

I like to prescribe it after my initial 5-week treatment with my first-choice supplements, especially in cases where the Candidiasis is present mainly in the esophagus, ear, nose or throat. However, with the appearance of a more active and safer medication (DiFLUCAN) in 1990, Nizarol has lost a lot of its attraction.

* Capryllin (GRL)

Scientific literature has long indicated that Caprylic acid should be effective in killing candida albicans. Capryllin (GRL) responded to that demand effectively. It is formulated as a time-release preparation. The coating of Capryllin allows for slow release of Caprylic acid along the entire length of the gastrointestinal tract.

Start with *one* capsule with meals, three times a day, for three days. Continue with three tablets, three times a day, for the next five days and finish with four capsules, three times a day, for two weeks. Then, go to a maintenance dosage of two tablets twice a day for one month at least, after which time each patient must be evaluated individually. *Always* take Capryllin with meals, since it is an acid and as such can cause stomach pain and gastritis. It is not unusual that the maintenance dosage has to be continued for at least three months.

One of the advantages of Capryllin is that it is available in health food stores and is rather inexpensive. However, conduct this therapy only under the guidance of your doctor.

* DiFLUCAN (Fluconazole)

With the appearance of Diflucan ™, all other anti-fungal medications have taken a back seat. In a study done by the Division of Infectious Diseases, at St. Pierre University Hospital, Brussels, Belgium,the effectiveness of Diflucan was compared with Nizarol and found to be twice as effective and much less toxic for the liver. (2)

Excellent results are seen with Diflucan to combat the yeast aspect of CFIDS patients. You will notice a couple of other differences from Nizarol.

* First of all, its price: A 200 mg. tablet of Nizarol costs about $2 a tablet. Diflucan comes in 100, 200 and 400 mg tablets. You need to take 200 mg daily, and a 200 mg tablet costs about $9! If you do this as a sole therapy, you must finish a three-month course. Insurance mostly reimburses.

* Onset of die-off symptoms. While Nizarol will cause die-off symptoms (explained in Chapter Twelve) within the first week, Diflucan seems to trigger these symptoms in the third week. It is important for you to recognize and prepare yourself for these symptoms. Otherwise, you might conclude wrongfully that you are getting worse.

It is important to keep in mind that not all drugs will work the same for every patient. While some patients experience rapid relief, others get better more slowly. It is important to work with your doctor to get sound advice during the course of your treatment. Don't expect a miracle cure from drugs alone. The miracle of peak immunity comes about when you follow the rules of healthy eating and boost your immune system.

* Homeopathic Herbal Products

This is the most revolutionary and effective method I have encountered for the thousands of patients I have treated. This method is the future therapy, the most efficient and extremely fast-working. It is the number one treatment in my office, and it is the safest, most cost efficient and most efficient of all the treatments discussed before. It is discussed in Chapter Ten.

* Replace the Normal Flora:

The normal intestinal flora comprises three parts. The main flora consists of Anaerobe bacteria (Bacterium Bifidus and Bacteroides). The secondary flora is composed of the E. Coli,

Enterococci and Lactobacilli. The third contains Yeast Cells, Clostridia and Staphylococci.

Billions of these friendly bacteria (L. Acidophilus and Bifido bacteria) are essential in order to inhibit the growth of yeast cells. Normal flora can be destroyed after only a few days with antibiotics and need to be replaced in order to avoid the creation of a favorable environment for the yeast. By supplementing your daily diet with stable, high potency L. Acidophilus and Bifido bacteria, you are greatly enhancing your body's natural ability to keep dangerous and/or pathogenic micro-organisms under control. And replacing the normal flora is absolutely necessary after treatment of candidiasis to prevent a relapse.

There are many people who would benefit greatly from using L. Acidophilus supplements, but who feel that they cannot successfully do so due to lactose intolerance or other milk-based allergies. They reluctantly purchase so-called "hypo-allergenic" or "milk-free" products that claim to be superior in potency and viability due to the absence of milk in their processing methods. However, what the public is not aware of is the fact that by not culturing their microorganisms in a milk base, the viability and potency are severely impaired.

Lactose-intolerant patients do not manufacture "lactase," which is a naturally occurring enzyme whose function is to break down milk sugar into a more simple form which the body can then digest. However, by introducing very small amounts of a high-quality acidophilus product, you can stimulate the natural production. Then the body will begin to take care of this function on its own. Therefore, the optimum way to conquer milk-based allergies is to introduce various strains of acidophilus bacteria into the system in small increments (1/16-1/8 tsp once daily) and gradually increase these amounts weekly to the minimum recommended dosage of 1/2 tsp daily.

Looking at all the brands available on the market, you might be confused. One of the best products available is Lactobacillus liquid and Lactobacillus capsules (non-dairy) from GRL. The normal dosage of the liquid is 1 Tbsp after each meal, or one capsule after each meal. This product is also excellent for vaginal yeast infections - douche with 1 Tbsp Lactobacillus in 3 ounces of water for several evenings.

* As its taste is close to that of yogurt, acidophilus is a favorite preparation to give your children in case of constipation or other gastrointestinal disturbances.

* Make sure you don't fall into the trap of buying cheap, fruit-flavored acidophilus brands. These are less concentrated and therefore inferior to the Lactobacillus mentioned above.

* It's important to remember that once you open a bottle of acidophilus (powder, capsules or liquid), you must keep it in the refrigerator to preserve the quality of the viable microorganisms in it.

Failure to restore proper flora in the gut will inevitably lead to relapses of yeast overgrowth, no matter what medications are taken to kill these yeast cells. So far, the products on the market, mainly the Lactobacillus products, sometimes mixed with bifida bacteria and bulgaricus, yield mixed results.

* Who should take acidophilus?

If you have an immuno-suppressed condition such as Candidiasis, CFIDS, AIDS or a viral condition such as herpes simplex, taking acidophilus is a must. It should be taken automatically when antibiotics are administered, either orally or intravenously, to counteract the inevitable yeast overgrowth and/or reactivation of latent viruses. Women with vaginal yeast infections or urinary tract infections should use acidophilus diluted in water as a douche to clear infections. In addition, they should take it orally to prevent recurrence of infection.

Gastrointestinal disorders such as gastritis, stomach-and duodenal ulcers, Colitis Ulcerosa and Crohn's disease will benefit from a restoration of the normal intestinal flora. In fact, looking at the causes of immuno-suppressed conditions, acidophilus can be taken as a preventive measure by everyone, children included.

Now that we've covered some of the methods for treating viral illness and candidiasis, as well as CFIDS symptoms, the next chapter will launch you on the path to continuing good health. It's called "Seeking the Best Therapy: Conventional vs. Alternative Treatments."

REFERENCES:
(1). "A Randomized, Double-Blind Trial of Nystatin Therapy for the Candidiasis Hypersensitivity Syndrome," William E. Dismukes, M.D., et al., *The New England Journal of Medicine*, Vol. 323, No. 25, December 20, 1990; pages 1717-1722.

(2). "Comparison of Flucanozole and Ketaconazole for Oropharyngeal Candidiasis in AIDS," De Wit, Geerts, Goosens and Clumeck, M.D.s, Division of Infectious Diseases, St. Pierre University Hospital, Brussels, Belgium, *The Lancet*, April 8, 1989, pages 746-747.

CHAPTER TEN

SEEKING THE BEST THERAPY:

CONVENTIONAL VS. ALTERNATIVE TREATMENTS

Ellen P. was desperate when she consulted our office. After a year-long search, she had found a doctor who could establish a correct diagnosis of CFIDS. But Ellen still felt fatigued, bloated, constipated and unable to perform her regular accounting job. Her concentration and short-term memory were still severely affected. Her doctor had tried Prozac ™, Sinequan ™ and Zantac ™, all with little effect.

The initial relief of finding the right diagnosis had now been lost in despair of finding an available and effective therapy. What was the point, Ellen wondered, of being labeled as a CFIDS patient, if she still felt as bad as she had before? It was not until Ellen changed her diet and started to receive homeopathic injections for her underlying and ongoing yeast infections that her symptoms started to recede.

This chapter describes some exciting therapies which can help you just as Ellen P. was helped.

By now you have some idea of the diagnostic tests your doctor should be ordering for you. Once you know what you have, the next logical step is to treat the underlying condition, whether it be reactivation of a virus, overgrowth of yeast, or invasion of parasites.

Everyone who has CFIDS will benefit, too, from the peak immunity diet described in Chapter Eleven. But trying to boost your immune system before the underlying condition is treated is like jogging barefoot to the athletic shoe store: you'll keep incurring damage along the way until your immediate problem is addressed. After six weeks of treatment for your underlying condition, you can start boosting your immune system with the supplements outlined in Chapter Thirteen.

In Chapters Four through Eight, different medications for the sub-diagnoses (parasites, yeast, viruses), were discussed. In this chapter, you will learn about the preferred treatments for yeast, viral and parasitic involvement in CFIDS patients, as well as a description of conventional medical treatments.

Look to Ancient Views

Reduce Stress

After taking the self-scoring questionnaire and learning about the triggering factors for CFIDS and related conditions, you can begin to grasp the kinds of environmental and lifestyle changes imperative for your improved health. Common sense can be your guide when you look at the present stresses in your life. Evaluating your emotional and personal directions is imperative if you expect to get well and stay well.

Old Remedies Offer New Approach

One of the pitfalls of modern interventionary medicine is the ever-present side effect. The practice of medicine becomes a balancing process: weighing the possible harmful side effects against the potential cure of the drug or therapy. Often such a choice is made because doctors and patients want immediate results, and are willing to worry about long term side-effects later. The consequences are often serious — millions of people addicted to sleeping pills and painkillers, or suffering degenerative conditions as a result of chronic cortisone therapies.

Aside from these health consequences, medications are expensive, draining the coffers of the family, producing resentment, sadness and despair. AZT, hailed as the only helpful medication for AIDS (in spite of its side-effects), is a prime example of this: one year's course of the drug costs about $10,000 (although now it is more like $5,000 because researchers found that half of the initial proposed doses of AZT works as well), which would be staggering even for a well person to pay for. Inexpensive, effective and safe medications are needed for debilitating conditions such as CFIDS, candidiasis and viral illness.

That's where homeopathy and acupuncture come in. With people increasingly reacting to the artificial preservatives used in prescription medications, a pure and natural art such as acupuncture has a lot of value for the immuno-suppressed patient. Acupuncture has been shown to increase the production of T-Helper cells and increase the activity of phagocytes, as well as improve endocrine and hormone function. These qualities are especially helpful for someone whose immune system is deficient.

Homeopathy, which relies on natural treatments, was created by Dr. Samuel Hahneman, one of Napoleon Bonaparte's doctors. On his route to conquer most of Europe, Napoleon used the innovative skills of Dr. Hahneman to keep his troops free of typhoid fever. Hahneman's new concept of medicine, which he called "Homeopathy," derived from the Greek words, "homeos," which means "similar," and "pathos" or "disease." Hahneman's basic law was, "Let's cure a disease with the disease itself, or "Like cures like."

Hahneman's theory still has an enormous following in Europe. In France, Belgium and Holland, you can find thousands of medical doctors trained in homeopathy. In the United States, its popularity has suffered because of policies by powerful medical associations, pharmaceutical companies, potent medications and exciting laboratory techniques.

How Homeopathy is Different

There are major differences between homeopathy and conventional medicine.
* For one, homeopathy rarely has side effects; conventional medicine almost always has.
* Homeopathy is affordable, while conventional medical treatment can be very expensive.
* Homeopathy treats the patient in a way that supports the immune system, whereas conventional medicine often blocks the natural defense mechanisms (cortisone being a perfect example).
* Homeopathy treats the cause; conventional medications often treat only the symptoms (think of anti-fever and anti-rheumatic medications).

Relying on Hahneman's original ideas, homeopathy considers symptoms to be the body's defensive reactions. The homeopathic practitioner uses therapies that program the body to heal itself. In conventional medicine, the doctor may prescribe medicines that counter what is happening, often hampering the body's natural defense system. The diagnosis in homeopathy largely depends on a painstaking inquiry, often as long as two hours, where physical *and* mental symptoms are taken into consideration.

Modern medicine all too often views the mind and body as two separately functioning entities, to be treated by different doctors, observing and respecting the body-mind unit. Therefore, the object of homeopathic treatment is a permanent resolution of the condition, and more and more doctors are turning to its methods to treat immune-suppressed conditions.

What Are Homeopathic Injections?

Developed by Hahnemann, homeopathic treatment is based upon the "law of similar," which held that the power of a drug to cure a disease is related to its ability to produce symptoms of the disease itself. However, Hahnemann also believed that the body's healing mechanisms could be triggered by very small doses of a drug, or combinations of drugs. And that is precisely what is used in homeopathic modern treatments: herbal products, diluted in homeopathic doses, leaving behind spirit like substances that set in motion the body's "vital force" or QI.

Hahnemann wrote: "*For as far as the greatest number of diseases are of dynamic (spiritual) origin and dynamic (spiritual) nature, their cause is therefore not perceptible to the five senses. Homeopathic medicines act upon our well-being wholly without communication of material parts of the medicinal substances, thus, dynamically., as if through infection. Far more healing is expressed in a case in point in the smallest dose of the best dynamized medicines, in which there can be, according to calculation, only so little of material substance that its minuteness cannot be thought and conceived by the best arithmetical mind, than by large doses of the same medicine in substance. That smallest dose can therefore contain almost entirely only the pure, freely-developed, conceptual medicinal energy, and bring about only dynamically such great effects as can never be reached by the crude medicinal substance itself taken in large doses.*"

Homeopathy is the use of minute doses of drugs that bring on symptoms similar to the disease to stimulate a cure. For example, it is possible to dilute an aqueous solution of an antibody indefinitely without the solution losing its biological activity. Strangely enough, at some dilutions the activity falls off; on further dilution, it is restored.

The combination of herbal supplements in a homeopathic dose, injected in acupuncture points, is not only a completely safe treatment, but also the most efficient one. The beauty of this approach is that it is completely natural. In Europe, ancient arts of medicine, such as acupuncture, herbology and homeopathy, have been incorporated into modern therapeutic modalities with great success. Injections of vitamins or herbs into carefully selected acupuncture points have been performed in Holland, France and Germany for years with good results.

An excellent study showing the effectiveness of homeopathy was published in the prestigious British medical journal, *The Lancet*, on October 18, 1986. "Is Homeopathy a Placebo Response?" (Ref. 1), showed "that patients taking a homeopathic preparation showed a greater improvement in symptoms of hay fever than those taking a placebo; this difference was reflected in a reduced need for antihistamines, increased in significance when adjusted for pollen count and time of season, and was confirmed by the doctors' assessments."

A similar study was performed by Ferley, M.D., et al.: "A Controlled Evaluation of a Homeopathic Preparation in the Treatment of Influenza-like Syndromes." (Ref. 2) The researchers reported that the proportion of patients with influenza who recovered within 48 hours of treatment was greater among the homeopathic treatment group than the placebo group.

In June 1988, the British journal *Nature* published a study that supports the homeopathic theory. In the report,"*Human Basophil Degranulation Triggered by Very Dilute Antiserum against IgE*", (Ref. 3), a French allergist, Jacques Benveniste of the University of Paris-Sud, found that white blood cells, basophils, react to an antibody solution after the equivalent of 120 tenfold dilutions. Up to 60% of the basophil membranes were disrupted by these weak solutions. It was as if these homeopathic solutions remembered their earlier larger concentrations. The publishers of *Nature* were so startled by these results that they waited two years before publishing them. The homeopathic researchers were confident enough with their results that they announced that they would do controlled studies. The second team, visiting Dr. J. Benvenistes' lab came to a totally different conclusion. They found that the claims made by this doctor were "based on experiments which were ill-controlled." In the medical community, there is still a lot of skepticism about homeopathy, but it is making gains in popularity among practitioners because of increasingly successful results.

Safety of the Treatments

Homeopathic treatments consist of herbal products diluted in homeopathic dosage (ranging from one part herbal extract to 10 parts of water, to one part herbal extract to one-octillionth of water), and injected into the body at acupuncture points. The dilution to homeopathic strength makes these injections safe for any age group and for the most sensitive patients. Homeopathic dilutions are so small that they cannot be measured by normal laboratory standards. Therefore, harmful side effects are non-existent and even the needle prick is no more painful than the insertion of an acupuncture needle.

Results of the Treatments

Often patients who receive these homeopathic injections feel an immediate reaction. Many patients report feeling a sense of well-being, a clear brain, a surge of energy and a feeling of being centered for the first time in a long while. Almost always, the next day a Herxheimer or die-off reaction (see Chapter Twelve) is experienced. The symptoms of this reaction, caused by the toxins leaving the body, may include headaches, flu-like symptoms and fatigue, often relieved after a good bowel movement. The die-off reaction might last for two to ten days, after which the patient feels a higher level of energy and clear headedness.

There are numerous advantages to this method. Besides the low cost and lack of side effects, this kind of treatment takes only a couple of months, where previous treatments for candida for example, with Nystatin, Capricin, Tanalbit, Nizarol or Diflucan, can take from three months to one year. The length of these treatments, coupled with the necessary dietary changes, can be quite discouraging for candidiasis patients.

The rapid results of homeopathic treatments allow patients to start adding in wheat, rye, yogurt and additional fruits to their diets as early as six weeks.

The speed with which we are achieving results is also very encouraging. Each treatment brings major changes when the patient follows the well-outlined program. After the initial die-off period, each week groups of previous symptoms decrease in intensity or disappear. It is very encouraging when the digestion starts working properly, when there are days that the energy level is up or when one can think clearly for the first time.

There is one caution to keep in mind when you receive homeopathic treatments. You may feel so energetic, free from attacks of dizziness and bloating, that you may be tempted to go overboard with certain foods too early in the program. The awakening is rude. Almost immediately, headaches, bloating, constipation and brain fog symptoms reappear. Fortunately, you can rebound immediately if you get back on track again.

During this cleansing period, you will be extremely sensitive to any bad foodstuffs you ingest. In fact, you will react with more severe symptoms to the same foods than during the period when you were really sick. Don't be alarmed by the die-off reaction symptoms. It is simply your body telling you: "Don't add this junk to me while you are in the process of cleansing me."

Length of Treatment

Injections are given in a course of five treatments, with a seven-day interval between each injection. Following this major part of the therapy, there will be a follow-up visit after a three-week interval. More frequent injections might be required depending on the individual case, because each case of CFIDS is different.

Follow-up by a well-trained physician is absolutely necessary in order to make changes during the course of the treatment. It is obvious that the patient will have to adhere to a healthy life-style in order to boost the immune system, once the viral and candida titers begin to drop.

What Herbs Are Used?

Yeast-Fighting Herbs

There are many fungus killers present in nature. These include Pau D'Arco (discussed on page), and Australian Tea Tree Oil or **Melaleuca Alternifolia.**

Virtually unknown in the United States, tea tree oil has a long history as a natural remedy. Widely used by the Australian Aborigines, the oil is a naturally occurring safe, powerful, broad spectrum antiseptic and fungicide. It has a pleasant odor and is non-toxic, as well as non-irritating to normal tissue. The oil is distilled from the leaves of Melaleuca alternifolia, a tree species which grows in the remote and rugged bush swampland of the north coast of New South Wales and the south coast of Queensland. It was named by Joseph Banks, a botanist who joined Captain Cook in his first explorations of Australia. Banks learned from the Aboriginal people that a delicious tea, to which they attributed powerful medicinal and tonic effects, could be brewed from the leaves of certain trees.

The use of this antifungal has been known for quite some time in Europe. A study done by Dr. Paul Belaiche, head of the Phytotherapy Department at the College of Medicine of Bobigny (Paris) showed that tea tree oil was active against Trichomonas vaginalis and Moniliasis. This was confirmed by another study done by Eduardo Pena, M.D., F.A.C.O.G. of Argentina in 1961, published in the *Journal of Obstetrics and Gynecology*, here in the United States.

Melaleuca has a powerful germicidal and anti-mycotic (anti-fungal) action which is very well tolerated by the vaginal mucous membranes when applied vaginally. It therefore allows a lengthy course of treatment which leads to the eradication of candida.

Herbs to Treat Viruses

The herbs used for EBV and herpes simplex viruses are similar in nature. Dioxychlor and hydrogen peroxide can both be used as single agents or combined to fight these viruses. Other herbs with known anti-viral properties are Rheum Palmatum, Forsythia suspensa, Centella, lomatia dissectum and Isatis tintoria. Use of these viral products will decrease the intensity of frequency of viral attacks.

Other Drugs Used for CFIDS Patients

Prozac

Depression is one of the biggest consequences of CFIDS. So it's no wonder that Prozac, an antidepressant drug approved in 1987, is one of the most-prescribed medications for this condition. Its action increases the amount of the neurotransmitter serotonin. Hailed for its lack of side-effects originally, it made even the front cover of a national magazine, *Newsweek*. Since the popularity of Prozac was largely hinged to its relative lack of side-effects, doctors started to prescribe it for the slightest emotional distress.

And then came a report from Harvard psychiatrist Martin Teicher, published in the *American Journal of Psychiatry*, showing a dark side of Prozac. Patients taking Prozac could become suddenly and obsessively suicidal. The recent scare stories have served a useful purpose, dampening some of the initial ecstatic claims about Prozac and prompting physicians to be more vigilant in monitoring their patients for severe mood swings and suicidal tendencies.

Although no prescription drug is absolutely safe, Prozac has its place in treating CFIDS patients. However, the time for starting this therapy should be more debated. For instance, when CFIDS patients start their treatments with diet changes and antifungal or parasitic medications, they will experience die-off reactions, as discussed earlier. Part of these die-off symptoms are depression, mood swings and suicidal tendencies. The duration of these symptoms is usually short-lived (1-2 days), so medications such as Prozac should not be necessary. If anything, patients are much better off taking a natural amino acid, Tyrosine, 1,000 mg, twice a day.

However, if the CFIDS patient becomes so overwhelmed by the emotional part of the disease, Prozac 20 mg daily, might be indicated. In this way, patients can use their energy to combat the physical part of the disease, while the emotional part is much better under control with Prozac. Caution should always be used, and medications must not take the place of psychotherapy.

Brain Fog Therapy

Brain fog is one of the more maddening symptoms in CFIDS patients. This usually shows up in the form of loss of concentration and short-time memory. Ensuring good bowel movements is crucial, because build-up of toxins can contribute to this symptom. However, some supplements, which are discussed in detail in Chapter Thirteen, can alleviate the intensity of this symptom. One of them is Germanium.

Another brain "stimulator' is *lecithin*. Lecithin is found in every living cell, and in highest concentrations in the brain, heart, kidneys and liver. In the brain, the lecithin choline will be transformed into the neurotransmitter acetylcholine, a vital component for the transmission of messages from one nerve to another. You can imagine how a lack of this transmitter can influence the memory and thinking abilities. The surprising finding in case of lecithin was that it was transported directly through the "blood-brain barrier." In other words, it goes easily from the bloodstream into the brain centra and tissues, something that is difficult for many other medications.

This means that each time you take lecithin there can be an immediate effect on the production of neurotransmitters in your brain. Do we need to supply our diet with lecithin? For CFIDS patients, a resounding "yes", and older people too, since there are few significant dietary sources. Depending on the brand, 2 capsules daily of lecithin will work adequately as a brain tonic.

Ampligen: The Drug of the Century?

Ampligen is not a new medication. It is an immuno-modulatory and anti-viral agent that was used 10 years ago in a number of cancer trials. In spite of increasing the production of interferon, the drug had to be stopped because of its toxic side effects (bone marrow toxicity). However, scientists developed a process that transformed ampligen into a substance whose half-life is approximately 20 minutes, which means that the immune system does not have time to form antibodies against it. After initial favorable test trials done by Dr. Peterson of Nevada, four sites were selected for FDA-approved drug trial for the treatment of CFIDS: Incline Village, Nevada; Charlotte, North Carolina; Portland, Oregon; and Houston, Texas. The initial results showed improvement of participating patients in their IQ performance levels. Unless the statistical analysis shows that patients receiving ampligen show marked improvement over the "placebo: patients, the study will go on for a while and FDA approval is still miles away.

What are the cons of ampligen? Its cost is estimated at about $2,000 a month! No small feat for most CFIDS patients who already have spent thousands of dollars on extensive tests and fruitless therapy. Side effects such as nausea, insomnia and flu-like symptoms have been noticed but these can be due to the Herxheimer or die-off reaction as described in Chapter Twelve. A major mistake I see is that CFIDS patients taking this drug will think of it as the typical "magic bullet," taking care of all their needs, forgetting about triggering factors discussed in Chapter Two and diet and life style changes, discussed throughout this book. I was shocked to see at a recent CFIDS conference, where speakers were praising ampligen, that coffee and sweets were served to the CFIDS participants. I cannot understand this ignorance. But if ampligen will at least improve some of the facets of CFIDS, it is my sincere wish that it would be availabe to everyone, not just to a small portion who can afford it.

Once your physician has determined that you are sick with CFIDS, candidiasis, viral illness or AIDS, you need to get treatment for that underlying condition. This chapter has dealt with various mainstream and alternative remedies. The next chapter tells you how to get the right foods for peak immunity, so that you can avoid relapses.

REFERENCES

1. "Is Homeopathy a Placebo Response?," David Taylor Reilly, McSharry, Arrchison, M. Taylor; Glasgow Homeopathic Hospital, Dept. of Bacteriology and Immunology, University of Glasgow; *The Lancet*, October 18, 1986,881-885

2. "A controlled Evaluation of a Homeopathic Preparation in the Treatment of Influenza-like Syndromes," Ferley, J.P., et al., *British Journal of Clinical Pharmacology*, 27:329-335, 1989.

3. "Human Basophil Degranulation Triggered by very Dilute Antiserum against IgE", Benveniste et al., Universite de Paris-Sud, Clamart, France; *Nature* Vol. 333 30 June 1988.

CHAPTER ELEVEN

EAT YOUR WAY TO PEAK IMMUNITY:

SEVEN PRINCIPLES OF HEALTHY EATING

Principle #1: Making the Decision to Eat Well

Americans are obsessed with losing weight. Almost every bookstore has several shelves filled with the newest books on losing weight. Despite the proliferation of commercial weight loss centers and a hoard of diet formulas, most people find themselves in the "yo-yo" syndrome: losing several pounds, only to gain them back when they resume their normal patterns of eating.

We all know that overeating is not good. The media tell us so; the American Heart Association and American Cancer Society do too. Why, then, is it so hard for people to make real changes in their eating patterns?

A diet is restrictive. And when people feel deprived, they cannot keep up a routine that continues this deprivation. Although the trend is now changing, many fad and commercial diets put too much emphasis on limiting calories and not enough on good nutrition.

To be successful and really help people, an eating plan needs to take into consideration the whole person. "Dieters" should be encouraged to examine all the aspects of their lives, not just how many calories they're taking in. People have to learn to identify the factors that trigger overeating. They may need to learn how to use their leisure time, how to handle job and relationship stress, how to develop exercise habits. In support groups like Overeaters Anonymous (OA), people learn how to pinpoint the triggers for their overeating. When they can learn to deal with those, healthy, nutritious eating will follow.

Why We Overeat

We don't eat just to satisfy physical hunger. The act of eating is loaded with social and emotional implications. This is not new, of course. Throughout history, human beings have used meals as a way to celebrate and mark important cultural and personal events. But eating to satisfy emotional hungers works against good health.

There are many groups of emotional eaters. Those who eat to escape depression are the most prominent. For these people, food provides a great comfort. When family or friends are critical or disappointing, relief through food is always available. This idea may have started with the person's parents. These messages are also reinforced by the media. When it's cold and rainy outside, and you had a hard day at school, what's more comforting than coming home to homebaked cookies and milk? The unfortunate reality, of course, is that the relief from food is short-lived, and that you must keep feeding that emotional appetite. The foods you eat may give you a momentary "high," but the letdown is worse, adding extra pounds and guilt to the original depression.

Eating the Wrong Foods

Perhaps you don't eat too much. Some people who are quite slim have another problem — eating the wrong foods. We all know that "junk food" is bad for us. But it's still hard to switch to good food. Why is this? Most people perceive "health food" as tasteless, colorless and having strange texture.

Health food is none of those things. In fact, it suffers from a bad reputation. We perceive health food as bland or strange because our taste buds have been programmed to expect the salt-fat-sugar flavors. It is possible to retrain your taste buds, however. Have you ever omitted sugar from your diet for a time, and then tried to eat your favorite candy bar? Often it doesn't turn out to be the treat you thought it would be. The same is true of salty foods. When you become used to foods that are either unsalted or lightly salted, you can immediately taste the overuse of salt in restaurant and frozen foods.

Food Controversies

You may already be eating healthy food. But then you run into other problems: health professionals can't seem to agree on what constitutes a healthy diet. The cholesterol controversy is a prime example. Years ago, people ate a lot of fish, eggs and meat. Then eggs and fish fell into disgrace in favor of the Omega-6 fats of deep-fried foods. But after a 1984 Harvard medical study about the eating habits of Eskimos, fish such as salmon and halibut, which contain omega-3 fats, were recommended again.

The latest item to cause confusion for consumers is oat bran. The "cholesterol-lowering effect of oats" got especially high marks, even in highly respected medical magazines such as *The Lancet*, a British medical journal, (1) and *The American Journal of Clinical Nutrition* (2). Then a 1990 study published in *The New England Journal of Medicine* concluded that oat bran was no better than plain white flour when it came to lowering cholesterol levels. This put a damper on sales of oatmeal and oat bran products. However, only 20 people with relatively low cholesterol levels were involved in the study.

These controversies do not instill confidence in consumers. Certain people may conclude, "Why bother? If the experts can't make up their minds, we might as well eat Twinkies, chocolate bars and apple cakes today, because we can expect that some expert might decide that these are healthy tomorrow."

There are other sources of confusion in the field of nutrition. Today many people know more about the link between diet and disease than the typical physician did in the 1970s. But much of the awareness comes from food advertising, not from health professionals, a fact which results in continuing confusions about the specifics of the diet-health link. That may be one reason that people still do not understand the difference between cholesterol and saturated fat in food. When choosing foods that are less damaging to your heart, you should examine the *saturated fat* content rather than the cholesterol content. Polyunsaturated oils such as corn, sunflower and safflower are healthful, so long as they are consumed in moderate quantities. Mono-unsaturates, such as almond, olive, avocado and walnut oil, are the most healthful.

Food Labeling Problems

There are no laws governing food labeling in this country. While many foods do contain the nutritional information on the label, descriptive terms are not regulated. This means that you have to be extra careful when you choose foods in the market. Current food labeling policy evokes some urgent questions. Should health-related claims about food be regulated? Should food labels provide better nutritional information? The answer to these first two questions is certainly yes. What are the responsibilities of food companies? They should be to give us descriptive food labels that are not misleading.

For instance, terms like "light" and "natural" are used on labels to signify that they are light in fat or calories. But these terms are not defined by the federal Food and Drug Administration (FDA). The term "light," for instance, may refer to the texture of the product — light and fluffy — or to the color of the food. A typical example is cooking oil where one can actually see that some oils are lighter in color than others. Although such oils are often labeled "light," they may not have a lighter fat content.

Another eye-catching label is "high fiber." Yet, "high fiber" is not defined by the FDA either. As a result, it can appear on foods that contain less than two grams of fiber per serving. The RDA, or Recommended Daily Allowance, of fiber is five grams.

Although there are no reliable standards for food labeling now, there are groups who are lobbying for standards in labeling. One of these is the Center for Science in the Public Interest, based in Washington, D.C. Their newsletter, *Nutrition Action*, is an excellent source of updates on food labeling and additive controversies. To obtain it, call (202) 667-7483 or write to:

> Nutrition Action Health Letter
> Circulation Department
> 1501 16th St.
> Washington, D.C. 20036-1499

What Is Organic?

Organic means "grown without the introduction of chemical pesticides and chemicals." Since the scare in '89 with alar-tainted apples and the continuous threat of grapes loaded with pesticides, America's interest in chemical-free food has been stronger than ever. After years of struggling for recognition and acceptance, the organic food industry is experiencing more popularity. Organically grown food is now considered mainstream. More growers are experimenting with this environmentally sensitive process and are looking for alternatives to conventional farming with its reliance upon chemicals to combat mold and soil quality problems.

But is food labeled "organic" really what it says? And according to whom? To the average customer, organically grown tomatoes might look suspiciously like the regular tomato in the next store on the street. Ideally, to ensure that you're getting truly organic food, you would have to grow it yourself. That's no small feat, given our crowded time schedules and availability of land.

The most practical thing to do is educate yourself and ask questions of your grocer. If there is no certification label on the box, ask your grocer to produce it. It might also be interesting to know when produce can be called organic. A farm must be chemical free for at least three years before its produce can be called organic, as defined by most organic certification programs, such as CCOF (California Certified Organic Farmers), the OGBA (Organic Growers and Buyers Association of Minnesota), NOFA (National Organic Farmers Association of New York), and the Texas and Washington State programs. Anything less than that, as certain California growers try to introduce, is NOT acceptable.

The first principle of eating for peak immunity involves a conscious decision on your part to eat well. That's not easy, given all the messages to be slim. And once you resolve to eat well, you'll encounter other hurdles: conflicting advice from health professionals, misleading food labels, and foods that may not be wholly organic. With some research and the help of this book, though, you can make the changes and achieve peak immunity. It takes perseverance and courage to adhere to a healthy eating plan. But once you've started on the path, the rewards of more energy and a better self-esteem are immeasurable.

REFERENCES:

1. DeGroot, a.P., et al. "Cholesterol-lowering Effects of Rolled Oats." *Lancet*, 1963: volume 2, pages 303-304.

2. Kirby, R. W. et al. "Oat-Bran Intake Selectively Lowers Serum Low-Density Lipoprotein Cholesterol Concentrations of Hypercholesterolemic Men." *American Journal of Clinical Nutrition*, 1981: volume 34, pages 824-28.

Principle #2: Avoiding the Diet Traps

No matter what food plan you ultimately choose, some additional elements have to be present if you're going to succeed.

Flexibility

Does your selected plan:
> * Allow you to eat away from home? This could become increasingly difficult if restaurants don't change the way they do things.
> * Allow you to eat foods you like and give you healthy and tasty recipes for newly introduced foods?
> * Offer a regimen low in sugar and fats, and high in complex carbohydrates and protein?
> * Encourage exercise and teach new eating habits, mostly through behavior modification techniques?
> * Achieve these goals safely and inexpensively?
> * Promise long-lasting change and NOT a quick fix?

If you answered "no" to just one of the questions above, chances are that the food plan will let you down in the long run. You need the flexibility in lifestyle changes to really make your new eating plan "stick." Keep searching.

Common Sense Rules

Once you have found a diet-program that will work for you, the following common sense rules will be applicable. Whether you are being treated for an immuno-suppressed condition or are simply trying to boost your immune system, you will be given specific eating guidelines by your holistic doctor. And at the end of this chapter, sample food lists are provided.

* Chew food thoroughly, 20 times for each mouthful. Digestion begins in the mouth with the enzymes in your saliva. Most immune-suppressed conditions (CFIDS) have some relation to malabsorption. In this syndrome, the digestion is so poor, that the body's cells cannot draw nutrients from the food, leading to toxicity, obesity and sluggishness.

* Drink liquids between meals, not with meals. Drinking liquids during meals will dilute your digestive juices.

* Eat only in the dining room and with the rest of your family if possible. Dinner has to again become a feast where manners are observed and joys are shared.

* Don't skip meals. Many people think they are making the right move by skipping breakfast and sometimes lunch as well. The

result is a lazy digestive system that lacks the continuous stimulus provided by food intake. "Night-eating syndrome" leads to burning fewer calories. Breakfast is especially easy to omit, but the word breakfast should remind you of what it really is: "breaking the fast" from the previous night.

* When emotionally upset, eat less; the digestive chemistry is changed, preventing complete digestion. In reality, most people will stuff themselves when upset, drawing them in a spiraling movement of depression and physical discomfort.

* Keep a brief food-related-symptoms journal of everything you eat or drink to learn more about how specific foods affect your disposition and health. Record them over a period of time and use the diary to spot problems.

* Avoid distractions such as TV, radio or reading while eating. These activities will distract you from focusing on chewing thoroughly and maintaining the relaxed mental state which assists digestion and nutrient absorption.

* Read labels and ingredients on boxed, canned and packaged foods.

When dining out, ask questions about the ingredients used in preparing your food. Be prepared to be assertive. Some waiters will not communicate these small wishes to the kitchen. They may think, it's only another health nut making my job difficult, when you say, "I can't have any sugar, MSG, soy sauce, or preservatives."

Often waiters think they can ignore such requests because you won't even notice it. Yet anybody, suffering from candida, CFIDS or other malabsorption syndromes, can react severely to these substances. I know of one CFIDS patient who gets the waiter's attention by telling him that the last time she ingested MSG, the restaurant had to send her to the hospital! You may not feel comfortable being this dramatic. Some people make little cards mentioning the foods they have to avoid and hand them to their waiter at the appropriate time. This allows you to avoid having to go through your whole litany and the waiter will probably remember it better.

* Use proper food combining. See page 154 for additional information.

* Eat only when you are hungry. The average person eats for many reasons, most of them the wrong ones: because it is 6 p.m.; because they are upset; because they happen to be together with

friends and eating is a wonderful form of communication and entertainment.

A longer space between meals will enable the digestive system to recuperate from the last meal. Enzymes can be produced in enough quantities to allow effective digestion. Most of us could eat breakfast and dinner, without having to snack in between and be perfectly happy.

* Stop blaming someone else or something else. You've probably heard the following excuses yourself (or maybe even used them yourself!): "My husband does not support my efforts to lose weight," "I had all that food in my refrigerator and I could not let it spoil," and the all-time favorite, "I have no time to shop for this health food and no time to prepare it."

It doesn't require that much more time to make a healthy meal than to prepare junk food. Another favorite target is your doctor who prescribed this "stupid diet" which "does not allow you to eat anything." The ultimate responsibility for our eating habits and our health is ours and ours alone.

* Last of all, remember: there are no quick fixes, only permanent ones through the modification of behavior.

By incorporating these common sense rules from principle #2 into your eating plan, you'll be making your own success a lot easier to achieve. Changing your eating patterns is an ongoing process and you must be patient and forgiving with yourself. Being too hard on yourself is a sure way to feel worse. Most people go in stages when they change eating habits. If you feel you have to first leave out the worst elements in your diet before you reach the peak immunity diet, then do it!

Principle #3: The Secret of Food Combining

I often hear my patients say, "Why am I not losing weight? Why am I still bloated and uncomfortable after eating, even when eating the good foods? I am eating less than my friend who has weird eating habits, yet he never has a weight problem and seems always to have plenty of energy."

Such references to weird eating practices are often really references to food combining. Food lists and calorie counts are the two aspects of dietary health that are most frequently stressed. Food combining is not. This is a practice based on the nutritional discovery that certain combinations of food are digested with greater efficiency than others.

Food digestion consumes more energy than any other function of the human body. The increased requirement of blood supply to the digestive system can deplete the brain's oxygen, making you sleepy in the early afternoon. Only food that is completely broken down by our enzymes will be absorbed by the blood and transferred to our cells. CFIDS patients, especially, must adhere to food combining rules, since they all suffer from malabsorption, caused by yeast overgrowth or parasite presence.

Let's take a typical American lunch or dinner: a baked potato, a steak, vegetables, followed by a fruit dessert. Consider what happens during this meal. The steak requires an acid digestive juice (hydrochloric acid) to break it down. But the baked potato, eaten during the same meal, requires an alkaline one. It does not take a scientific brain to see that the acid and alkaline digestive juices will neutralize each other, giving a signal to the body to produce more juices, since digestion is incomplete. But the newly produced juices are again neutralized. This repetitive effort by the digestive system in generating enzymes can lead ultimately to its exhaustion. In the meantime, as a result of being in the stomach too long the meat has putrefied, while the starch from the potato contributes to the bloating, gas and discomfort, because it has had time to ferment.

To make matters worse, many people top their meal off with a "healthy" fruit desert. This compounds the problem. Fruit can be absorbed by the body directly, so the long digestive process is bypassed. Indeed, watermelon, apples, oranges, cantaloupe, grapefruit, peaches and prunes pass through the stomach in less than an hour, compared to the two hours required by other foods. If you eat fruits for dessert, they stay in your stomach longer than they should. This creates even more fermentation and putrefaction, requiring a large expenditure of energy to push the mass into your small intestines. Once there, another 24 hours are required for it to travel through the intestinal tract. Are you still surprised that you feel bloated, gassy, seven months pregnant and dead tired at 2 o'clock in the afternoon? In such a state, it is surprising that your brain can work at all.

To modify your current diet to create proper food combinations, you must remember that different foods require different lengths of time to be broken down. Here are some basic tips to remember when planning your menus:

* Fatty foods are the most difficult for the body to digest. Fried foods, gravies, rich sauces, pastries, shrimp, ham, pork and

bacon may require up to five hours for their breakdown into smaller compounds. Can you imagine what havoc you will create in your stomach if you eat these goodies with your veggies and fish?

* For proper digestion, one protein at a time is the golden rule. Different proteins require different enzymes for digestion, so don't combine cheese, for example, with chicken. The different digestive enzymes required for their breakdown in the stomach may cancel each other out.

* Melons should be eaten alone: they digest so easily that they proceed directly through the stomach, faster than any other fruits. Combining fruits, such as apples and pears, will hold them up for an unnecessary amount of time, causing extensive fermentation.

So, by following principle #3, the secret of proper food combining, you're allowing your body to use energy more efficiently. You'll feel the difference! Consult the food-combination chart below for more information.

Figure #9 shows the food-combination chart.

Principle #4: Coping with Cravings

Anyone who suffers from candidiasis and/or CFIDS knows that cravings can rule their life. There is an irresistible urge, a driven feeling for the body to consume certain foods. What do these cravings mean — do they fulfill certain basic physiological needs? And how can you cope with them when they happen to you?

Causes of the Cravings

In an article entitled, "Does Your Body Know What It Needs? Cravings," (*Good Health Magazine*, the *New York Times*, September 27, 1987), various opinions were expressed: "There is no physiological reason to explain these cravings." (Dr. Richard Mattes, Monell Chemical Center in Philadelphia); "These foods are craved because their consumption will either satisfy a nutritional deficiency or, particularly with carbohydrate cravings [attention Candidiasis-sufferers!], serve as a form of self-medication to counteract depression." (Dr. Judity Wurtman, Biochemist at the Massachusetts Institute of Technology)

Other opinions included the following: "Carbohydrate cravings are linked to people with seasonal depressions and therefore, what they have crave is actually what they need." (Dr. Norman Rosenthal, psychiatrist at the National Institute of Mental Health).

FOOD COMBINING CHART

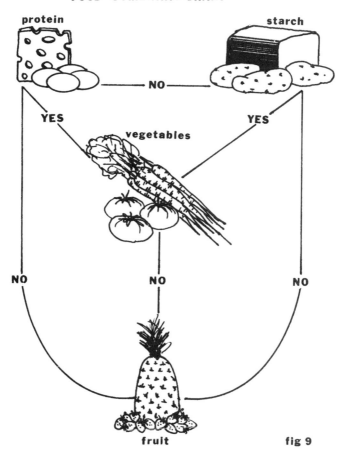

fig 9

By following the lines between food groups, you can see whether you should combine these foods at one meal. Example: by starting with protein and following the line down to fruit, you'll see "no" along the line. This is because fruit will not be digested as quickly, and will ferment in your digestive tract, if you eat it with protein.

Women do report food cravings more often than men, most likely because of food desires related to menstruation and pregnancy, according to Dr. Harvey Anderson, Chairman of the Department of Nutritional Sciences at the University of Toronto Medical School. He found that carbohydrate consumption increases by 30% just prior to menstruation.

Another study conducted at Kansas State University by Katharina Grunewald, Associate Professor of Foods and Nutrition, found that most women in the study craved chocolate more during menstruation than at any other time of the month. Cravings for popcorn, potato chips and hamburgers were not increased by the menstrual cycle. She states: "We don't know why women crave more chocolate during the menstrual cycle, we simply know they do. It may be that they want to do something pleasant for themselves."

Recalling Chapter Two, you may remember what the Chinese believed about food cravings. Their belief was that when we crave a certain taste (sweet, salty), the organ belonging to the taste was suffering. The spleen-pancreas is suffering when we crave sweets and other carbohydrates (CBH). So to some extent it is true that their consumption will satisfy a nutritional deficiency: the *moderate* consumption of CBH (if at all possible — extreme cases of Candida/CFIDS will not tolerate this at all) and sweets will strengthen the spleen-pancreas. However, when patients experience cravings, they are not talking in terms of "moderate amounts." Usually the patient can get on a roller coaster of sugar intake, having quite the opposite effect of what we are discussing. Consumption of sugar or CBH will improve their mood for only a very short time (half an hour). Afterwards, inevitably, they will collapse with severe mood swings and depression.

Women with yeast overgrowth often also have PMS and experience severe cravings for CBH, especially sweets, in the week or so preceeding their menstrual periods. The reason for this is simple. Progesterone levels increase before the menstrual cycle leading to increased glycemia (sugar) in the blood. Yeast cells respond by multiplying faster, sensing the presence of increased sugar. So it is simply the *yeast cells'* cravings. What a mistake, though, for these patients to follow the advice of Dr. Rosenthal, who claims that what they crave is actually what they need! As countless candidiasis sufferers will attest, this increased sugar intake would lead them, more probably, to more mood swings and depression.

Dealing with the Cravings

The first step is to recognize cravings for what they are: signals to warn you to eliminate the food or taste that you're craving. Easier said than done, you say. Well, there is some help available:

* Acupuncture has certain points that can cut the cravings immediately, even before you make adjustments to your diet.

* **Carnitine**, an amino acid taken in tablet form two to three times a day, can cut your cravings too. This is usually sufficient to get you past the initial cravings.

* **GTF Chromium**, which helps regulate the sugar-insulin balance, can be very helpful if taken twice a day.
* **Green Magma**, 6 tablets a day before meals.

Even if patients are tempted by some sweets, many are surprised to discover that these sweets no longer taste "as good as they used to." The basic idea of principle #4 is this: recognize the craving for what it is, and then work to curb it. Natural help is available, as you will see with the food choices lists later in this chapter.

Principle #5: Increase Energy and Avoid Mood Swings

You can do this quite naturally by selecting the right kinds of foods. In fact, you can manage the food you eat to alleviate disturbing symptoms such as insomnia and morning fatigue, as well as depressions and mood swings. As you can imagine, not all foods will be able to give you these quick positive changes in mood. As explained earlier, the Candida/Peak Immunity diet is a high-protein, low-carbohydrate one. This is just what the doctor ordered for your symptoms.

Protein for Energy

If you are suffering from CFIDS or Candidiasis, eating protein will increase your energy in the morning, avoid the post-lunch doldrums and bolster your energy throughout the day. But don't go right out and eat steak! Not all protein will have the same effect. The most effective energy boosters will be the proteins low in fat: fish, shellfish, veal, chicken without the skin and *very* lean beef. For healthy people not suffering from Candidiasis, low-fat milk and low-fat yogurt will have the same effect.

Carbs for Calm

If you want to achieve a calming and more relaxing effect, one that will reduce anxiety and let you fall asleep more readily, carbohydrates are in order. There are two types: the sugars (glucose, sucrose, fructose and lactose) or the starchy carbohydrates (potatoes, corn, and vegetables).

Food and the Brain

Eating more protein will boost your *energy*, while eating more carbohydrates will calm you down and sometimes make you sleepy.

Why is this? Small chunks of information are transported from one brain cell to another by means of chemical substances, called *neurotransmitters*. There are two classes of these chemicals manufactured by the brain from the foods we eat: the "alertness" chemicals (Dopamine and Norepinephrine) and the "calming" chemical Serotonin. Tyrosine is the amino acid from which Dopamine and Norepinephrine are produced. Serotonin is produced from its precursor, *Tryptophan*. These two amino acids will enter the brain with other essential amino acids. Tryptophan is known for its calming effects. Eating foods rich in that amino acid will help you calm down. And the converse is true of the proteins which break down into the amino acid Tyrosine. You'll get a "kick" from ingesting foods high in that amino acid.

If you are suffering from Candidiasis or CFIDS, you should eat proteins at breakfast and lunch, when you need the energy. Then eat carbohydrates at night with little protein, to ensure a calming effect.

So you see, that principle #5 is simple: it is *not* a matter of luck to feel energetic and happy. If you use the information in this principle of eating well, you can modify your moods and help your suppressed immune system get better.

Principle #6: Know Your Fats

"Total cholesterol," "HDL and LDL," and "Saturated fats" all have become household words. Why, with all this information blasted at the public, do people still have problems in selecting and preparing foods that reduce the risk of obesity and heart disease? Conflicting messages on food labels may be one reason. Ignorance about possible food "time bombs" may be another. You don't need to go back to school to take extensive courses in nutrition and biochemistry. Simply knowing the differences between saturated and non-saturated fats will contribute more to a low cholesterol count, than avoiding cholesterol rich foods altogether.

Simply put, saturated fat is fat which will become solid at room temperature, like butter or bacon grease. Your local American Heart Association office is a good source of free booklets and pamphlets on eating for a healthy heart.

Unlikely Sources of Fats

For a long time, many of our favorite cookies, crackers and breakfast cereals were made with highly saturated tropical oils such as lard, coconut oil and palm oil. So by eating your favorite snack, you were possibly clogging your arteries with cholesterol deposits. Why these saturated fats? Because they account for the crunchiness and freshness of our cookies, a fact the American public insists on. However, that is changing, due to the large amount of media attention to the dangers of high cholesterol levels.

The big food companies had to make adjustments. So they promised to get rid of all these saturated oils and replace them with more healthful unsaturated ones, corn or canola, for instance. End of the story? Unfortunately no. Torn between the public's demand for delicious goods and the cholesterol ban that swept the country, cookie producers did the only thing they could do: they saturated the unsaturated fats, a process called "hydrogenation." Companies could still advertise they were health conscious by using the unsaturated fats, and still produce our heavenly snacks just the way we wanted them. What they forgot to mention is this: soybean oil, probably the most common hydrogenation candidate, is increased in saturated fat percentage when it is partially hydrogenated. That's not the only bad news. Hydrogenation transforms unsaturated fats into "trans fatty acids." These fatty acids are stable and solid and therefore look AND act like the dreadful saturated fatty acids.

So, as the customer, you need to be aware of the term, "partially hydrogenated"; it is a red flag to your good health. Processors are not required to say anything about the trans fatty acid content, leaving the gates wide open to misinformation for what healthful foods should stand for. It sure looks like we can't have our cake and eat it too.

Which to Pick?

What are we to do? Fat is fat, but it wears several different hats. Many people still believe that because they use margarine instead of butter, non-dairy creamers instead of milk and polyunsaturated fats, they are on the path to a healthier diet. Yet, margarine is a synthetic substance, produced by processing vegetable oil, but then hydrogenated to make it solid. This way, an unsaturated fat is transformed into a saturated one. Still, it is better to pick a margarine that has twice as many polyunsaturated fats as saturated ones. For instance, a label showing you five grams of poly-unsaturated to two saturated, points you to the most healthy margarine. Non-dairy creamers, loaded with fats and polyunsaturated fatty acids, do lower the total cholesterol, but have at the same time the unwanted effect of lowering HDL, our beneficial cholesterol.

What's left, I hear you ask?

* Avoid these saturated fats if at all possible: the ones found mainly in cheese, lard and meats.
* Omit the tropical oils such as coconut, cocoa butter and palm.
* Avoid hydrogenated products.
* Concentrate on the mono-unsaturated fatty acids such as olive, sesame, walnut, cashew, canola and avocado.
* Choose the "extra virgin" olive oil. This term describes the highest quality oil with the best flavor, color and aroma. It is produced in smaller quantities than other grades and is priced the highest. Oil that does not meet the standard for virgin oil is refined to remove impurities, then blended with virgin oil. This blend is labeled "pure" olive oil.

Other necessary changes to reduce fats in your diet include:

* Broil, poach or steam instead of frying.
* Increase the amount of vegetables, fruits and beans you eat. They will increase the amount of complex carbohydrates which will help reduce blood cholesterol and calories.
* Limit cholesterol-rich foods such as egg yolks and organ meats (liver, etc.).
* AVOID: Lard, bacon fat, mayonnaise (unless the better ones in healthfood stores), French fries, fried foods, hamburgers, salami, hot dogs, caviar, pork, poultry skin, croissants, doughnuts, milk shakes, chocolate, sour cream, whole milk, cream cheese, potato chips.

Is it all worth your trouble? You bet it is. In countries where animal and fat consumption is limited, and the diet is comprised of cereals, grains and vegetables, the incidence of heart disease, cancer, obesity and diabetes is rare. We really have met one of the greatest enemies of this century—and it is fat. Too many people have already dug their graves with their forks and otherwise intelligent people shorten their lives by ingesting fat as if there were no tomorrow.

Principle #6 is really quite direct: recognize the harmful fatty foods and replace them with low-fat alternatives. It's the best guarantee of your future good health.

Principle #7: Avoid the Trigger Foods

The preceding principles have given you basic rules for food choices. All you need to know now is what foods you absolutely should avoid and which ones you can introduce right away. The list of the foods to avoid and the ones to introduce is not cast in stone.

For CFIDS and Candidiasis patients, it's best to adhere strictly to this foodlist until you sense a real increase in energy. Depending on the rest of the therapy you do, you could reintroduce foods as fast as five weeks after starting your diet. But this should be an individual choice: you first have to feel better before you will do the next move. Even then, introduce one food at the time, so that you can monitor your reaction to that particular food. If you are introducing three foods at the time, and you feel bad one hour after that meal, there is no way for you to find out to which one of the three you reacted.

While these food suggestions are imperative for CFIDS and Candidiasis patients, anyone who has food allergies, who wants to lose weight in a sensible way or who simply wants to increase his or her energy, should try this diet for five weeks. Five weeks is the amount of time that will allow you to feel better, because you have stopped feeding this problem (yeast/parasites) or eliminated allergic food factors from your diet. When you are feeling more energetic, it is much easier to stick to healthier food habits and I hope that these 5 weeks are only the beginning of a change towards lifelong commitments to eating healthier.

Forbidden Foods

You might think, at first glance, that some of these foods belong on the "good" food list. Some of the foods are on this list because they are fermenting foods (apples, pears, grapes, wine, beer, champagne, vinegar, tofu, soysauce) and others because they feed a particular problem in the patient (yeast-containing foods, such as breads, wheat, rye, mushrooms and dairy products). Others such as red wine contain sulfites (asthma sufferers watch out!) and urethane, which appears naturally during fermentation. Urethane is a chemical, long recognized to cause cancer in animals, which causes concern about its effects. Even when you are not a CFIDS or Candidiasis patient, you will greatly benefit from omitting these food stuffs. The majority of the population has maldigestion and malabsorption and avoiding these foods will greatly enhance the power of your digestive system.

THE FORBIDDEN FOODS LIST

* Breads: including yeast-free wheat and rye breads. However, rice and corn breads, unleavened and ponce breads are fine.
* Dairy products: except butter, eggs and goat's milk, goat's cheese and yogurt; other yogurt from cow's milk is not allowed.
* Mushrooms, wine, champagne and beer or anything else that is fermented, such as miso and tofu.
* Fruits: especially not apples, pears and grapes; also no watermelon, cantaloupe, oranges, peaches, prunes, dates or dried fruits (too much sugar).
* Wheat and Rye: in crackers, cereal, breads and pasta.
* Salt: use sea salt if needed. Absolutely no sugar in any form; avoid Aspartame (Nutrasweet, Sweet-N-Low), no honey, molasses or maple syrup.
* No tea or coffee, not even caffeine-free coffee, or herbal teas; exceptions are mentioned further. No fruit juices except the juices of allowed fruits; even then, use them sparingly; and certainly do NOT use fruit juices when fasting.
* No tomato or barbecue sauce (unless you make your own without peppers, sugar, vinegar, syrup).
* Avoid raw and cold foods (except salads occasionally; more about salads is discussed later). Remember, these foods decrease the strength of your digestive organ, the spleen-pancreas as outlined in Chapter Two.
* Absolutely no vinegar: in salad dressings, use mustard and mayonnaise.
* No oatmeal, for at least four weeks.
* No horseradish, peppers.
* No canned foods or fried foods.
* Avoid refrigerated left-overs, especially meat; freeze the left-overs and heat them up later (this is especially the rule for meats, since they will become damp and moldy overnight).
* Avoid ice in drinks.

After reading this list, you might think that there's nothing left in your refrigerator that you CAN eat. Don't despair. Consult the "Good Food List" below.

THE GOOD FOOD LIST

(It's a good idea to rotate foods to achieve variety and to eliminate allergies and sensitivities.)

Fruits: Papaya, mango, kiwi, pineapple, banana, honeydew melon, coconut, guava, grapefruit, berries and lemons. Eat in the morning at breakfast. Do not eat after meals. About 10% of patients will not be able to eat fruit at all because of the high fructose content (such as in bananas) or because of high acidity (pineapples). CFIDS patients should eat fruit sparingly during the first four weeks on the program.

Juices: Water with lemon juice; fresh-squeezed vegetable juices; unsweetened cranberry juice; wheatgrass juice; fruit juices of allowed fruits (in moderation); coconut milk.

Grains: Brown rice, wild rice, millet, buckwheat, amaranth, quinoa, popcorn, corn tortillas, corn chips, "polenta," teff

Brown Rice Derivatives: Mochi, brown rice syrup, rice cakes, rice crackers, riz cous, creamy rice, "Rice and Shine," "Creamy Rice" brown rice cream (a hot cereal), rice dream beverages (almond, carob)

Beans and Legumes: All beans are allowed, including garbanzos, humus, lentils, black beans, pinto beans, etc.

Meats: Chicken, turkey, veal, lamb and rabbit.

Fish: The National Academy of Sciences and the U.S. Food and Drug Administration (FDA) report on low- and high-risk seafood varieties. Tuna generally has low levels of environmental contaminants. Cod, pollock and haddock are found in deep offshore waters, also making them low in chemical contaminants. Ocean-caught salmon is notorious for parasites and should be fully cooked to destroy worms and amoebas, but is otherwise free of contaminants.

Canned tuna is rarely a cause of food-borne illness unless mishandled by food preparers. Beware of shrimp, though, because these scavengers of the sea are frequently mishandled in the store or in the home. As an extra precaution, consumers may want to reheat shrimp to destroy any possible bacteria or parasites. The greatest number of illnesses from fin fish come from the tropical varieties: mahi-mahi, bluefish, barracuda, grouper and tropical snapper.

Fresh water fish from the Great Lakes, such as whitefish, from Santa Monica Bay, from Puget Sound and the Chesapeake Bay may carry undesirable levels of chemical contaminants. Swordfish can carry elevated mercury levels and should be avoided, especially by women of child-bearing age.

The highest-risk seafoods are mollusks - oysters, clams and mussels - eaten raw. The intestines and viscera are the parts that we consume, and they contain all possible kinds of contamination, natural and man-made.

Dairy: Goat's milk, goat's cheese, goat's yogurt, butter and eggs. For those with high cholesterol levels, butter and eggs should only be eaten on an occasional basis. When you do this and leave out sugar and other foods on the "no" list, you will decrease your LDL (bad cholesterol) and increase your HDL (good cholesterol).

   Oils:

* Olive oil: use only organic cold-pressed, extra-virgin olive oil. (So-called pure olive oil or virgin oil are second-rate.)
* Sunflower and safflower oils: choose the unrefined high-oleic varieties of these oils for cooking and baking.
* Canola oil: the newest oil in the market is also the best. It contains linolenic acid, the Omega-3 fatty acid that reduces blood cholesterol levels and prevents clogging of the arteries.
* Other allowed oils are avocado, sesame and flaxseed oils.
* *Nuts, Seeds, Nut Butters and Nut Milks:* (Store in freezer or refrigerator) All are allowed except peanut and pistachio products. *No peanut butter!* Nuts, seeds and nut butters should be eaten in moderate amounts, since they contain high amounts of calories, especially fats. For instance, one handful of cashews equals 750 calories. Keep in mind that roasted nuts are easier to digest than raw ones.

Vegetables: Steam or stir-fry all vegetables; avoid eating them raw. It is all right to have lettuce with fresh tomatoes and avocadoes and a salad dressing consisting of an allowed oil with lemon juice. Sundried tomatoes are also allowed.

Seasonings, Spices, Herbs & Condiments:

* Quick Sip by Bernard Jensen (a tamari-like sauce)
* Bragg's Liquid Aminos
* Garlic, Onion, Sea salt (sparingly), dill, thyme, tarragon, rosemary, oregano, curry, basil, parsley, paprika, cinnamon, nutmeg, carob, etc.

Beverages:

* Pau D'Arco tea, water, water with lemon juice, peppermint and spearmint tea (excellent for digestion), Uvi Ursa tea (great for urinary tract symptoms and to help strengthen the bladder)
* Other herbal teas (without caffeine) to be used sparingly. Watch out for either dryness or mold content, if they are stored for long periods of time.

Breads: Don't forget, bread has yeast and sugar, so you should avoid breads for the first four weeks of the eating program. Then incorporate them very slowly into your diet. Here are some of the breads you can choose:

* Ponce whole rye (wheat and yeast-free)
* German sourbread (wheat and yeast-free)
* Rudolph's 100% rye bread with linseed (also wheat and yeast-free)

As you can see from this list, you won't go hungry when you eat well. The best way to make good food choices is to think about what you eat, read the labels, and keep the Seven Principles of Healthy Eating in mind. Using these principles to guide your eating patterns will enhance your immunity and sense of well-being. Therefore, adhering to these principles will help with AIDS, EBV, Candidiasis and other immune-depressed conditions.

CHAPTER TWELVE

"IF I'M GETTING BETTER,
WHY DO I FEEL WORSE?"

Cindy T. was eager to start following her doctor's advice. After all, she had suffered from CFIDS for 10 years and felt hopeless after numerous failed therapies. For the first time, a complete change of diet was suggested, a diet that was high in protein and low in carbohydrates. Together with antifungal medications, the diet treatment offered Cindy a glimpse of hope about her illness. After only three days on the new treatment, Cindy phoned her doctor. She felt overwhelmed with fatigue and joint and muscle pain. She felt betrayed to be feeling these symptoms after rigorously following her doctor's advice.

How can it be, you may ask, that Cindy is feeling worse after she began eating better? It's a lot to ask of someone to give up the foods they love in favor of healthier foods. And it's only natural to expect a payoff in terms of feeling better. But feeling temporarily worse should not be interpreted as a bad sign. When you switch to higher quality foods, you can expect to experience the onset of new, and not necessarily improved, symptoms.

As you saw in the preceding chapter, the Peak Immunity diet is based upon choosing protein-rich quality foods. The closer food is to its natural state, the higher its quality and the better it is for you. Nuts and seeds, eaten in their natural state (i.e., not roasted or cooked in oil and salted), are superior to chicken which, in its turn, is superior to beef. The quality of a nutritional program is also improved by omitting toxic substances such as coffee, tea, chocolate, tobacco and salt.

"Okay," you say, "I'm willing to give up junk food and eat these high quality foods." Are you expecting to feel an immediate and obvious improvement, as well as a sense of well-being and relaxation of your anxieties about your health? Then you need to be prepared: this is not going to happen overnight. Yes, you can get better and stay healthy by altering your eating habits. But it took a long time to get where you are now, and the body will not heal itself without first discarding lower-grade materials and making room for the higher quality ones.

What you must remember in the first challenging weeks is that you are offering your body alternative materials to the toxic substances (coffee, sweets, fried foods, etc.) which we sometimes find so tempting. This is the time to "hang tough" with your eating program. Do not be tempted to abandon it because of the symptoms you may be experiencing. These are completely normal. During the cleansing phase (the first weeks of the diet and the therapy you follow for candidiasis, viruses and parasites), the **HERXHEIMER** or **die-off reaction** will occur. Do not be alarmed, and do not quit your new eating program. The phenomenon of toxin build-up has been known for a long time and was described as early as the beginning of this century.

Dozens of medical papers from the past were devoted to the subjects of "*Chronic Intestinal Stasis*" or "*Intestinal Toxaemia*" (*Toxic Colon*). In the volume which recorded the 1913 proceedings of England's Royal Society of Medicine, 380 pages are devoted to the subject of toxin buildup alone. Sir W. A. Lane, Surgeon to the Royal Family of England, and one of the most eminent doctors of his day, spent most of his life trying to persuade his peers that many of the ills of modern man stemmed from "Toxic Colon." Here is a remarkable passage from one of these medical papers entitled "The Evolution of Disease" (*The Lancet*, Dec. 20th, 1919):

"The effect of auto-intoxication upon the brain and nervous system is very striking and calls for much sympathy. Headache, varying in intensity, is a common symptom. I have known it so severe, and accompanied with such violent attacks of vomiting as to lead a very distinguished neurologist to diagnose a cerebral tumor and to urge surgical interference. Neuralgias are frequent and may involve a great variety of nerves. They may be very intense. Rheumatic pains are constantly complained of. The patient, while sleeping badly, may find it difficult to keep awake during the day. Bad dreams are frequent. On awakening in the morning the feeling experienced may be that of extreme

prostration, no apparent benefit having been derived from the night's rest. The most distressing symptom of intestinal auto-intoxication is the depression which so frequently accompanies it. It varies in severity from a feeling of mental incapacity to one which not infrequently leads the sufferer to attempt to terminate an existence which has become intolerable. All efforts at mental concentration are futile, while any physical exertion is followed by a period of complete exhaustion...The term "neurasthenia" is very often applied to this condition of the nervous system...The patient loses control and fits of irritability or of a violent passion are not infrequent. Such a person is difficult to live with. Many are supposed to be stupid, dull, inattentive, or even imbecile.... The eyes are always affected. They afford an excellent and very delicate indication of the degree of auto-intoxication."

Sound familiar? This passage could be a textbook description of Chronic Fatigue or CFIDS.

Symptoms of Toxin Buildup

The following are some of the symptoms of toxin buildup. These will be different for different people. Toxins in your body will settle in various organs and systems. When you notice these or similar symptoms, tell your doctor about them. He or she may be able to suggest remedies for the die-off reaction, which is a necessary and normal part of your healing process.

The Eyes Have It

The eyes are the best indicators of auto-intoxication, as Sir Lane called it. Accumulation of toxins in the body will often dull the eyes. When the body is cleansed, they regain their real strength and brightness. Your eyes can display other evidence of toxins. Some people experience a grainy feeling, almost as if there is sand in their eyes. Lenses can become murky, eyes will start tearing and burning, or feel completely dry. Your eyelids may feel sticky in the mornings and need to be cleaned, or may exhibit rapid twitching movements.

Look at Your Tongue

Another obvious indicator of toxin buildup is the tongue. The presence of toxins in the colon, liver, small intestine and kidney is reflected on the back part of the tongue. You may be advised to check your tongue first thing in the morning. A thick white or yellow fur on the back part of the tongue reveals you may be suffering from chronic fatigue or yeast overgrowth. This will disappear as you improve.

A Different Kind of Headache

Some of the most frequent symptoms are headaches and fatigue. You might say, "I already experience these." But the symptoms caused by a die-off reaction are different from those you experienced before therapy. You can easily distinguish a toxic headache and a toxin-induced drop in energy within a day of starting your therapy and improved diet. "It felt like a bulldozer had run over me," and "I felt a dull headache on the top of my head" are patient complaints which express the magnitude of these symptoms.

Emotional Symptoms

Another intense symptom can be depression, from moderate to severe. Mood swings are common. You may feel quite cheerful at ten in the morning, but depressed by two in the afternoon. A person can't get much sympathy from friends, spouses or doctors when exhibiting this kind of behavior which provides a strong basis for characterizing CFIDS as a "psychosomatic" disease.

Some CFIDS sufferers go to emergency rooms in the middle of the night with severe anxiety attacks. Yet, clinical and laboratory examinations will usually not show anything, so the patient might be sent home with a prescription for Valium to ease the anxiety. What is really happening is this: During the night, your body is virtually inert — you don't sweat, urinate or defecate. The toxins build up to an intolerable level, which can cause you to wake up in a state of panic. In such cases an expensive trip to the emergency room can be prevented by an enema or high doses of Vitamin C, which help the body to rid itself of these toxins.

Muscle and Joint Symptoms

Muscle and joint pains are also high up on the list of toxin buildup symptoms. Two areas are usually the hardest hit: the neck muscles and the lower back muscles. With these kinds of symptoms, it might seem logical to consult your chiropractor. But it is important for you and your chiropractor to understand that an adjustment will not hold until your body is rid of toxins. So you might want to delay the trip to your chiropractor until some of the underlying problem (often candida overgrowth) is resolved.

Another symptom — and an area of potential misunderstanding — includes feelings of "pins and needles" and numbness in the limbs. Because these symptoms are closely related to those of multiple sclerosis and other neurological conditions, they can lead to a misdiagnosis. Yet, frequently, these symptoms are yet another sign of intestinal poisoning. They occur as a result of toxin building.

Where Toxins Leave the Body

These symptoms can make you quite uncomfortable. You may feel discouraged about your treatment when they occur. But you must recognize these symptoms for what they are — toxins, or poisons, that are causing you the discomfort. They are indicators that your body is releasing the toxins and that you are, indeed, making progress. However, it sometimes helps to know more about where these toxins exit the body.

There are several bodily exits for toxins, each of them the site of distinctive symptoms.

* The most obvious outlet is the bowels. The passage of toxins induces anal itching, burning and green stools.

* Another exit is the skin. Covering the biggest surface of our body, the skin, containing pores, sweat glands, nerve endings and hair follicles, actively participates in the cleansing process. When toxins exit through the skin, rashes, and sometimes hard, painful boils appear. Using cortisone creams are no help and, in fact, their effect is detrimental since they push toxins back to the interior. Just use some moistening cream, and the painful boils will eventually melt like snow under the sun.

* The urinary tract is another exit. The release of toxins can cause a burning sensation and frequent urination. These symptoms can also be erroneously diagnosed as "cystitis." The consequences can be dramatic if this error goes unrecognized. Since antibiotics are the prescribed treatment and since doctors often start a patient on antibiotic medication before urinary test results come back, then the problem will be compounded. These antibiotics kill the friendly intestinal bacteria, to cause yet another problem: yeast infection.

* The vagina is another exit. Vaginal discharge is often toxin release. Once again, if a vaginal anti-yeast cream or suppositories is prescribed, the problem will be compounded. Dead toxins will not

be affected by these medications, and often an aggravation occurs because of the chemical irritation. This is a condition known as "burning vagina," or vulvodynia (See Chapter Four). Douching with baking soda, vinegar, liquid garlic, Pau D'Arco or an acidophilus solution will take care of this symptom, while an adjusted diet and *oral* anti-fungal medication will treat the root of the problem.

       * The nose and throat constitute still another exit. If your nose runs and you are coughing up green, yellow sputum from your lungs, these can also indicate a release of toxins. Often, antibiotics are given when these symptoms present, aggravating the underlying condition. How can you protect yourself? By asking the doctor to take a culture of the mucus, from your throat or productive cough and *not* taking an antibiotic before the doctor has seen the test result.

       * The oral cavity is another exit. Foul breath and the presence of a white-yellow fur on the tongue reflect the cleansing process.

Remedies to the Die-Off Process

Once you understand and recognize die-off symptoms, how can you deal with them? How can you promote the cleansing process?

Achieving Good Elimination

       * Supplements and enemas

The biggest relief from toxin buildup will come through good elimination of our stools. What constitutes a "good" bowel movement? Patients and doctors often think that if they have bowel movements every three days, this is the way their body functions. Holistic practitioners take a different view. It is not healthy to have toxins remain in your system any longer than necessary. Even having one bowel movement a day does not guarantee complete elimination of toxins. Defecation can be incomplete or strained. It will definitely be influenced by the quality of your diet.

A good rule of thumb is: if you have three meals a day, you should have three bowel movements a day. Self-help aids are available in any health food store: high doses of Vitamin C, a high fiber diet, Colonic Rinse, Perfect Seven, Swiss Kriss, acidophilus, Pau D'Arco tea, SF capsules, Psyllium husk and super dieters tea are just some of the more effective cleansers. Most patients will notice, however, that these herbal products only work for a limited time.

The best way to remedy this is to alternate them. Of course, it makes good sense to rely on diet and exercise for proper elimination, but often in the beginning of the cleansing phases, an additional herbal laxative will be required. Above all, never forget to drink plentiful quantities of water (up to eight glasses daily) — your body requires water to carry the toxins away.

The next obvious step after these remedies is to use enemas. Enemas are more effective when combined with one TBS garlic, acidophilus or Pau D'Arco in 3 oz. of water. However, I do not encourage them more than once or twice a week since they tend to make the bowel sluggish. Enemas, too, are limited in their effectiveness, since the elimination they induce from the large colon is only partial.

* Colonic Hydrotherapy

The best help anyone can get in eliminating poisons from the body is through colonic hydrotherapy, sometimes called a high colonic. In this procedure, a disposable tube is inserted into the anus, and a lukewarm water solution is irrigated into the whole length of the large intestine. The procedure takes about 45 minutes and is able to dislodge and carry toxins which have been lodged over the entire length of the colon. An enema, on the other hand, reaches only the lower part of the colon. The therapeutic goals of colonic hydrotherapy are to re-balance the body's chemistry, eliminate old impacted stool and bring a high concentration of antifungal substances to every area of the colon.

Colonic therapy has fallen out of favor in the modern age because it is more time consuming than taking laxatives. Once again, we are the victims of our lifestyles. Indication for colonic therapy starts with the recognition of the signs of colon imbalance: headaches, alternating diarrhea and constipation, bloating, abdominal cramping and weight gain.

Normal daily bowel movements do not rule out colon dysfunction. Even after the use of enemas and laxatives, large amounts of feces can still be expelled through colonic hydrotherapy. When properly used, colonic hydrotherapy is a lot more than just a simple irrigation, as an enema is. It will include analysis of the stool and the irrigation of the colon with various solutions such as Pau D'Arco tea, acidophilus and Lactobacillus solutions (mainly to help build up the normal intestinal flora). The irrigation solutions vary according to practitioners. The most common solution is tap water, since it causes only mild inflammatory changes. Others use soap suds or oil.

The side effects of colonic irrigation may include temporary symptoms of nausea and diarrhea, due to the increased reflux (flow-back) of bile in the stomach. There can also be a potassium loss from using tap water enemas. You can prevent this by taking 20mEq/L of potassium daily.

Fatigue is a common symptom the day following a colonic hydrotherapy treatment. So many toxins have been stirred up that you cannot evacuate them in the same day. Most patients will not have a bowel movement the next day, which is not a reason for concern. There is widespread belief that colon irrigations wash out the normal intestinal flora. First of all, this is *not* the case. Second, people suffering from immune-suppressed conditions have very little friendly bacteria left in their colon, if any at all. Thirdly, the colon irrigation provides an excellent opportunity to improve the bacterial balance by implanting Lactobacilli during the irrigation.

Colonic hydrotherapy should be on the list of recommended therapies for every healthy person, but it becomes a MUST with immune-suppressed conditions such as CFIDS. The energy level of CFIDS patients is directly related to the amount of toxins accumulated in the body. The notion that "Health starts in the colon" is thus a matter of primary importance!

How do you choose a reputable colonic hygienist? Write or phone:

> The American Colon Therapy Association
> 11739 Washington Blvd.
> Los Angeles, CA 90066
> (213) 390-5424

The well-respected Connie Allred is the president of the association.

Other Treatment Modalities

Other excellent therapeutic modalities in relieving the symptoms brought on by toxin release include:

* chiropractic adjustments (make sure to treat your yeast at the same time or you won't hold your adjustments),

* massage in all its forms, including deep lymph massage and
* yoga exercises.

So if you are feeling temporarily worse when you start your new routine, remember the word temporary. These symptoms do not last forever. Your body needs some time to get used to having the proper materials for healing itself. In the meantime, you can use the tips included in this chapter to ease your symptoms. This will allow you to continue on the right course of healthy eating and proper therapies, which will lead you to Peak Immunity.

In the next chapter, you'll find out about other ways to boost your immune system.

CHAPTER THIRTEEN

HOW TO BOOST AND SUPPORT YOUR IMMUNE SYSTEM

Every day, we are bombarded with advertisements for medicines that promise quick relief for cold and allergy symptoms, for digestive discomfort. Wouldn't it be great if you could find one single pill that would increase the strength of your immune system? As Americans, we often look for a quick and easy "fix" to our health problems. But there is no magic bullet that's going to boost your immune system.

You have to do that work yourself, with the help of your doctor. But the good news is, it can be done! With the diagnostic tests, eating programs and alternative therapies described in this book, you can be well on your way to better health. And if you're healthy now, it can tell you how to benefit from the support of immune system boosters.

This chapter is about improving the functioning of your immune system. By paying attention to triggering factors, internal and external, that can predispose you to illness, you can decrease your risk factors. The key is in identifying the trouble spots and dealing with them. Zero in on your emotional risk factors and take care of them. Learn about the supplements that improve immune system function and start taking them. Give yourself time to exercise, and you'll see the benefits in your physical and emotional health.

Of course, to embark on this peak immunity program requires a commitment to change. And it's not easy to give up the "goodies" to which you have become accustomed. As you have seen in the previous chapters, those are the foods that are literally making you sick. You can choose to make a real difference in your own health. And who is more deserving of such a choice than you?

Only a whole-person approach can create the degree of immuno-competence that you need to safeguard yourself against disease. This chapter contains some powerful tools that can be used by both healthy and sick individuals. I am confident that new studies will confirm what ancient practitioners knew: you can increase the strength of your immune system in a surprisingly short time through some simple but powerful changes in your lifestyle.

Emotional Support for Your Immune System

It is no coincidence that I start with the emotional part of the therapy. You may recall that in the self-scoring questionnaire, there were many questions about emotional events in your life. That is because your emotional and physical well-being are interrelated. There is no separating your emotions from your physical self.

Many studies have been conducted (and many more are yet to come) proving that thoughts and emotional states can affect the body's immune system. I see it daily in my practice. Once patients have gone through the original therapy of CFIDS, for instance, relapses occur only when their immune systems diminish in strength. These relapses do not occur after normal food intake or after physical fatigue, but invariably after an emotional trauma. Divorce, separation, death or serious disease suffered by a close family member is almost invariably what causes reoccurrence of symptoms.

Not only do emotional traumas cause relapses, they frequently are the triggering factor for CFIDS or other related conditions. Whenever I see a new patient, one of my first questions is, "When did you last feel good?" and immediately after, "And when did you start feeling bad?" You would be amazed to see that almost 100% of these patients experienced an emotional trauma just before the outbreak of the condition. This does not mean that emotional trauma is the sole cause of the condition, but it is probably the straw that broke the camel's back.

An emotional trauma is the point of origin for most patients. It might be divorce, an ex-husband's remarriage, an old boyfriend who comes to town, etc. Even a happy event — such as hearing about a friend who is finally expecting the baby she has been longing for, can and sometimes does, depress the immune system. The self-scoring questionnaire illustrates this well: it is any significant change, whether it be positive or negative, that puts you at risk for illness.

Visualize Your Way to Health

What can you do to help yourself through difficult emotional times? There are some tools to connect the mind with the immune system. Guided Imagery or Visualization is one such technique. This has been used extensively by professional and amateur athletes to enhance their performance. For instance, an athlete might rehearse the perfect combination of movements in their minds before they go out to the playing field. Reviewing, for instance, a tennis stroke in your mind, before actually hitting the ball, will give you confidence and a feeling of focus.

Just as an athlete visualizes the successful combination of movements and correct follow-through, you can visualize yourself becoming a healthy, more energetic person. The key is in relaxing your body, and focusing on positive images for yourself. There are several books and audio tapes available in bookstores.

There are other uses for visualization. In the M.D. Anderson Hospital in Houston, Texas, young cancer patients play video games where they have T-cells pictured on their screen, zapping the bad guys, the cancer cells. It is believed that visualizing their enemies and protectors may positively Influence the functioning of their immune system. You can use this same idea to visualize the invaders such as candida cells or viruses roaming through your body. This may be helpful especially at times when you get those cravings for sweets, for instance. Visualizing how those yeast cells reach out for that food and start multiplying, killing all your healthy cells around them, will help to overcome cravings. The "Autobiography of a Yeast Cell," in the Appendix, illustrates how you can give your enemy a face, in order to deal better with it.

Express Your Creativity

Combining fun and therapy to enhance your defense mechanisms can take other forms. Many people, for example, have experienced the beneficial effects of artistic expression during their recovery from cancer. By immersing themselves in something they love to do, they ease their pain and bring beauty back into their lives. To balance the loss of quality in life and grieving that comes with immuno-suppressed diseases, writing a book, painting sculpturing or playing a musical instrument are as important as any form of therapy.

Many former CFIDS patients report that periods of confinement proved to be the turning point of their lives. They had no choice: they had to slow down considerably because they had no energy left; they had barely enough energy to survive. The generative force that comes with creativity proves to people that they can not only fight for their survival, but also that they can have a full life after receiving treatment.

It is important for all of us to realize that we are in charge of our feelings; our minds do what we program them to do. We can either program ourselves with self-imposed limitations that keep us from reaching our full potential, or we can fill our minds with good feelings about ourselves. You have to love yourself before you can love anybody else. Since your mind seems to be at work all the time anyway, why not switch it to this positive mental program? It can be meditation, self-hypnosis or imagery; it all boils down to the same result; our minds become focused and take full control of our bodies.

Don't fall into the trap of negative self-suggestion, where you tell yourself that you cannot attempt anything new. Telling yourself repeatedly about your shortcomings destroys any talent that you may have. Telling yourself you are inadequate and worthless will work — but against you. If you imagine yourself more as a winner, before you know it, you will be one.

When you discover how great it feels to be a winner, to be in control of your body, you might also find out how very refreshing and comforting it feels to use the power of your mind. So set your goals, try to determine what you want to accomplish, and go for it. If you don't have a mission, your mind will be in chaos, unable to guide your body in reaching those goals.

It is a good idea to set realistic goals at first. If you are sick, set yourself reasonable goals, and focus on one stage at a time, such as "I will follow the new eating program and take treatments for this week." Then after you have completed that first goal, give yourself praise and set the next goal.

If you are feeling truly overwhelmed by your feelings, then you might want to consider consulting a psychotherapist. There may be unresolved feelings from your past that are holding you back in your present life. Although it is sometimes painful to examine one's psyche, it is a journey worth taking if you can get to know and love yourself.

Biofeedback Techniques Work

Biofeedback is another mental tool that can speed recovery. Biofeedback is routinely used for conditions such as migraines and stress, but it also has been applied in psychotherapy. Biofeedback centers are common at university research centers, where subjects are "wired" to a machine that measures such bodily responses as pulse rate and perspiration. Subjects are asked to listen to buzz words designed to trigger stress or calm, and then to watch the machine as it measures their response. Then, in subsequent sessions, subjects are taught how to change the initial response and bring the pulse rate back to normal by such techniques as deep breathing, mental imagery, etc. You can find out about these centers by calling or writing universities or teaching hospitals who often offer such programs to the public.

Seek Your Own Community

Positive imagery and biofeedback are two tools that every victim of CFIDS, candida, cancer, etc. can use. Support from family and friends is another positive mental aid. Alas, while cancer patients often find the support they need, CFIDS or AIDS patients are more often rejected because of prejudice, ignorance or simply misunderstanding.

Feeling isolated from their loved ones, not being taken seriously by their doctors and closest family members, these patients will often experience anger and depression. Friends and family may feel at a loss. They feel powerless to help the patient, and that in turn may isolate the patient further.

I believe that, more than the lack of medication or a bad diet, negative feelings will depress the immune system and are responsible for the many relapses we see in these patients. It is incredible how many relationships and marriages have been broken up because of a lack of understanding and sympathy with the victims of these conditions. It is essential to realize that if the body is going to heal, then **emotional and psychological support are crucial.**

It may be up to the patient to find a community of support. The first step is in finding a doctor who will perform the right tests and confirm an actual physical diagnosis. The second step can be to connect with others who are experiencing the same condition. Support groups for Herpes victims, recovering alcoholics and countless others have sprung up across the country. Hearing that others suffer the same symptoms as you can be reassuring and healing.

Dietary Boosts for the Immune System

While we sometimes have little control over environmental "food," at least we have control, if we wish, over our personal daily intake of food. Even so, you must stay informed to avoid such possible dangers to food as irradiation, preservatives, carcinogenic colorings or added antibiotics.

Are there foods that would help maintain the strength of the immune system? The promotion of long life and good health through diet is no longer supported solely by folk wisdom and pseudo-science. Since 1980, the National Cancer Institute (NCI) has advocated research into whether diet can protect people from cancer. And if these foods are protective against cancer, the ultimate destruction of our immune system, they may have similar beneficial effects on other immuno-suppressed diseases. Even though many of the NCI studies won't be finished for several years, the picture is already clear enough to conclude that ALL of us can benefit from dietary changes.

Shop at Health Food Stores

Have you tried to find foods that contain no preservatives, sugar, coloring substances, hormones or antibiotics in your local supermarket? This is nearly impossible. The best start you can make for your dietary changes is by shopping solely in health food stores. Many patients have no choice in this. They may already react strongly to any additives in their foods. But these people are growing in numbers. And in a market-driven economy such as ours, the consumer can make a difference. By demanding different and more healthy food products, you can actually change what markets offer.

The peak immunity diet in Chapter Eleven outlined an eating program to stimulate your immune system. If you're healthy now, your diet can be less restrictive than one for a candidiasis patient, although the principles are the same.

Supplements Fuel Your Immune System

In this section, I discuss the supplements required to support your immune system. "Superfoods" are often considered "super" because they contain essential elements such as beta carotene, selenium, Vitamin C, etc., all of which are antioxidants, the critical fuel for building your defense system.

* Fiber, A Neglected Nutrient:

Fiber is a broad term covering a complex mixture of many substances. Initially it was defined as roughage of plants remaining after the digestive process. Fibers now also include some substances such as pectins, gums and mucilages found in many fruits. Fiber is not absorbed by the body and thus is not defined as one of the essential nutrients, requiring minimum daily requirements. However, it is critical for moving the digestive process along. It helps the colon carry out waste products.

The American diet, despite the increasing awareness of fiber's benefits, is still abnormally low in fiber. The current RDA (recommended daily allowance) of fiber is 10 to 15 grams, equivalent to either one heaping tablespoon of bran or 75 grams of wheat meal. We should increase our intake to 30 grams of fiber a day, equivalent to two tablespoons or 200 grams of bran, depending on our size (larger individuals should consume more).

Media coverage of President Reagan's colon cancer brought out the role of fiber in protecting against that form of cancer. Fiber not only plays a role in the prevention of colon cancer, but is equally important in the prevention of atherosclerosis and increased cholesterol levels, two factors linked to cardiovascular disease in adults (Ref. 1). In addition, evidence is now showing up that young adults are developing atherosclerosis at an alarming rate. During the Vietnam war, autopsies were performed on young victims (18 year-olds), and to the amazement of pathologists, sometimes extensive atherosclerotic damage was found in their blood vessels.

American kids get an average of 40% of their calories from fat, and they have the artery scars to show for it. Look at the major part of kids' food intake: potato chips, cookies, white bread, French fries, red meat, colas, candy, ice cream, etc. No wonder early coronary disease is documented more and more in young accident, homicide or suicide victims; and it is in direct proportion to their cholesterol levels. While adults' cholesterol level should be below 230 milligrams, a cholesterol count of even 150 mg is considered too high for children. So please, parents, since the burden for preventing future heart attacks is increasingly falling upon you, add fruits, vegetables and cereals (without sugar) to the diets of your children.

An important benefit for CFIDS and diabetes patients especially is that high-fiber diets lower insulin requirements and help control blood sugar. This way, CFIDS patients can control their hypoglycemic attacks and — what will come as music to the ears — they also can regulate their weght. All these benefits were outlined in an excellent paper by Dr. Anderson at the University of Kentucky in Lexington (Ref. 2).

DIETARY SOURCES OF FIBER

Foods (in portions of 100 grams)	Amount of Fiber (in grams)
Almonds	2.6
Artichokes	2.4
Beans, White	4.3
Beans, Lima	1.8
Blackberries	4.1
Boysenberries	1.9
Bran	7.8
Buckwheat	9.9
Carob Flour	7.7
Coconut Meat	4.0
Cranberries, uncooked	8.7
Lentils	3.9
Madadamia nuts	2.5
Malt, dry	5.7
Millet	3.2
Onions, flaked	4.4
Pears	1.4
Raspberries	5.1
Rice bran	11.5
Kelp	6.8
Wheat Bran	9.1
Wheat, shredded	2.3

Source: United States Dept. of Agriculture Handbook

* Antioxidants: Safeguards of Cellular Health

Stress in all its forms harms you by altering your cellular environment through the production of highly toxic molecules which have been termed "free radicals." A free radical is any molecule that has an unpaired electron in its outer orbit. This disrupts the molecule's electron balance. Excessive free radical activity will damage cells. It is implicated in all the degenerative diseases of our century.

What is the source of free radicals? Your body converts food into energy through a process called "oxidation," because it uses oxygen. Sometimes, oxygen becomes a free radical because it will have an odd number of electrons in its molecular structure (the resulting free radical is called superoxide). This is not an immediate problem if the amount of free radicals is minimal, since your immune system can use them to destroy bacteria and viruses. But your body has difficulty adapting when large numbers of free radicals are present. Cellular damage and premature aging of the tissues can begin. Another common symptom of excessive free radical activity is inflammation, affecting the joints and spine and causing different forms of arthritis.

Substances like vitamin E, vitamin C, beta-carotene, selenium and zinc are called antioxidants because they can neutralize free radicals. A second class of antioxidants is the antioxidant enzyme. Examples are superoxide dismutase (SOD), methionine reductase (MET) and catalase (CAT). Many of the antioxidants are discussed below. You will learn their role in maintaining the strength of your immune system.

BETA-CAROTENE

Beta-carotene has always been considered a frontrunner in the defense of our immune system. What is this precious nutrient? It is the precursor of Vitamin A, a "Provitamin." While Vitamin A consumption has restrictions (it is one of the only vitamins that can be toxic in overuse), beta-carotene is safe. There is a security system: beta-carotene is converted to Vitamin A as it is needed by the body. Even taken in high doses, it is harmless. Yellow palms and soles of the feet are signs of overdosage of beta-carotene.

For a long time we have known the benefits of Vitamin A provided by beta-carotene: improved night vision, growth of teeth, nails and hair. But beta-carotene is one of the most powerful anti-oxidants. An NCI-sponsored study conducted at Harvard Medical

School suggested enough evidence that foods rich in beta-carotene reduce the risk of cancer.

Does this mean that you should run to the health food store and start supplementing your diet with this miracle nutrient? You should examine your diet first. Surveys have shown that most Americans do not receive the recommended levels of Vitamin A. Judge for yourself. Do you eat enough foods such as carrots, spinach, sweet potatoes, parsley, kale and collard greens? If not, you belong to the majority. Therefore, supplementing with extra beta-carotene, especially in light of its non-toxicity, is advised. Take 25,000 units of beta-carotene, twice a day.

Another supplement, Spirulina, has attracted attention in this context. Beta-carotene is a major component of this extract of blue-green algae. Besides beta-carotene, spirulina contains many other carotenoids. The functions of the latter are still unknown, but they probably work in a synergistic way with beta-carotene and Vitamin E, another powerful antioxidant. Many studies are still under way, but so far we may presume that beta-carotene will be a major soldier in our immune system.

A study, directed at Brigham and Women's Hospital in Boston, in 1990 by Dr. Charles Hennekens, found that "a form of vitamin A (beta-carotene) common in carrots and many other vegetables appears to reduce substantially the risk of heart trouble in people who already have coronary heart disease."

VITAMIN E FOODS GET AN "A"

Especially in urban areas, environmental pollutants abound. More and more young people are developing sensitivities to gasoline fumes, perfumes, building materials, gas, and polyester clothing. Since we cannot immediately change our environment, we can protect ourselves by taking vitamin E, a potent antioxidant, which has a proven ability to protect cell membranes against chemical damage.

Smokers and menstruating women should be especially careful to replace vitamin E. Since estrogen destroys vitamin E, and many women may be using birth control pills, many have depleted levels of vitamin E in their bodies. Those who live in smoggy urban areas will also benefit from taking extra vitamin E.

In a study from the Human Nutrition Research Center at Tufts University, Boston, it was found that vitamin E may boost the immune system of healthy older people. Only after one month, participants taking 800 mg of vitamin E showed a significant improvement in immune cell response in comparison with a control group. As an antioxidant, vitamin E disarms free radicals—highly reactive molecules produced when our body uses oxygen and which are responsible for the wear and tear of bodily tissues associated with aging.

Food is not really a good supplier. You can find Vitamin E in eggs, spinach and cold-pressed cottonseed oil. With the tendency to omit eggs from the diet because of the cholesterol scare, it does not look like the average American will get much of the 400 I.U. Vitamin E daily. In case of fibrocystic disease of the breast, a doses of 800 I.U. daily has been shown to remedy the condition in 80% of the cases. Chances of conquering fibrocystic disease increase when Evening Primrose Oil is added (4 capsules daily).

VITAMIN C FOODS

Linus Pauling, Ph.D. and Nobel Laureate, extolled the virtues of massive doses of vitamin C in fighting disease and strengthening the immune system. The medical establishment refutes his views and emphasize the risk of developing kidney stones.

However, by focussing on that particular effect, you can miss out a lot. There is nothing better than high doses of vitamin C for common colds. In the case of flu, your first reaction should be high intake of Vitamin C, 1 tsp. buffered C powder, every other hour. If you get loose stools as a result, decrease the intake.

Vitamin C is certainly one of the biggest aids in the treatment of CFIDS. A Vitamin C drip will boost these patients' energy and spirit until the rest of the treatment has taken effect. It is not uncommon at all for patients to take up to 25 grams of vitamin C, a far cry from the recommended RDA dosage of 500 milligrams. In any case, a minimum of 4-6000 mg is advised for anybody who wants to boost their immune system.

Don't forget the abundant natural sources of vitamin C as well: it can be found in citrus fruits, berries, potatoes, tomatoes, cauliflower, corn and sagopalm.

ZINC FOODS

It is known that the thymus, behind the breastbone, grows from birth till puberty. From then on, it will only shrink in size. Since the thymus is the production place of the T-cells, this will limit their number. By supplementing one's diet with 50 mg zinc, especially the orotate form, you can effectively bolster the thymus.

The American diet is commonly deficient in zinc. And it is the elderly who need it the most. Since intake of extra zinc can cause gastric discomfort, it is best to take it after meals. Natural sources of zinc are round steak, pork, pumpkin seeds, eggs and mustard.

COENZYME Q10

As with many other supplements first brought to the attention of the public, Coenzyme Q10 has been hailed as a miracle nutrient. It was discovered in the United States in 1957, by Professor Crane at the University of Wisconsin. Human testing began in 1963 in Japan; in 1974, pure CoQ was used in organized trials. While CoQ prescription has reached a level in Japan close to that of the top five drugs, it is still not widely used in the Western world. This has more to do with commercial than scientific reasons. It is an important "co-worker" of the enzymes that guide the complicated biochemical reactions in our body. Every functioning cell in the body will be influenced by the presence of Coenzyme Q10. A lack of it will make these reactions sluggish and the cells will function at a decreased rate, initiating an array of diseases. It has been found that immuno-suppressed patients have low levels of Coenzyme Q10. More over it takes its place with the antioxidants — Vitamin E, Vitamin C and Selenium — in protecting our cells against damaging free radicals produced during the normal oxidation process.

It would seem wise to add to your potential of "soldiers" about 60 mg Coenzyme Q10.

GERMANIUM

The existence of the element Germanium was foreseen by Dmitri Mendeleev, the Russian chemist who put together the periodic table of elements. Later on, Germanium received little attention until Dr. Kazuhiko Asai, PhD, who established the Coal Center Foundation in Japan, focused his attention on the presence of Germanium found in coal. He developed a process for removing the Germanium from coal, and started to use it first on himself to cure his chronic arthritis, later on other people to help them recovering from different ailments. Before that, Dr. Asai showed that germanium added to soils would enhance plant growth. Dr. Asai, who has since founded the Germanium Institute in Japan, has dedicated his life to bringing the world the medical benefits of Germanium.

If you are looking for the "real" thing, you had better check the labels for "organic" Germanium or Sesquioxyde Germanium. It is available in different forms; powder, capsules and ampules. Doses seem to vary according to the condition. For CFIDS patients, 250-mg daily are advised. If you take the powder, which will be the most economical, it is better to divide the doses over different times of the day. It is also beneficial to hold the powder under the tongue, since absorption in the blood will be enhanced.

Germanium provides the body with more oxygen, therefore giving the body the opportunity to fight disease by its own powers. As with the other immuno-suppressed diseases, an alkaline diet (more fish, grains and vegetables, and less meat) is basic. A well-balanced diet is the beginning point of any health plan.

POLYZYM 22

This is an original product from Germany, produced by MUCOS Pharma GmbH, bought in Germany under the name WOBE-MUGOS and Polyzym 022 here in the USA (GRL). It is composed of Trypsin of pancreas 40 mg, Papainases 100 mg and Thymus 40 mg. As one can see, it contains the enzymes of the pancreas (the immune organ) and Thymus, the training organ of the T-cells.

Polyzym 22 has been proven to be effective (to some degree) in many auto-immune diseases. These diseases run in bouts and are associated with a derailed immune system: Rheumatoid Arthritis, Crohn's disease, Bechterew's disease, Co-Multiple Sclerosis (M.S.) and others. What is the mechanism of these diseases? They are a consequence of the continuing existence of immune complexes. Immune complexes are by-products of a reaction which occurs when antigens, such as chemicals, viruses, yeast cells or bacteria, enter the body and are bound by antibodies.

Under normal conditions these immune complexes are neutralized and, shortly after their development, eliminated again. They become dangerous when they are not eliminated, which is the case in auto-immune diseases. Immune complexes are deposited in the tissue, damaging the host's own cells. These deposits occur in the joints (causing Rheumatoid Arthritis); in the kidney (causing Glome-rulonephritis); in the intestines (resulting in the pancreas (leading to chronic recurring pancreatitis).

High doses of Polyzym 022 have been used in treating these conditions (10 tablets, 3 times daily), bringing favorable results and not causing the side-effects of cortisone preparations, the first-line drug in these diseases. In many patients remissions of up to ten years have been achieved.

In light of its effectiveness, Karl Ransberger, the manufacturer of Polyzym 22, has started a protocol (a detailed plan for a controlled study) for AIDS patients. The results are not yet known. But Polyzym

022 definitely results in a quick neutralizing of common cold viruses, seems to be on its way to playing an increasingly important role in the defense of our immune system.

Making the Right Choice

Now that you've read about all these wonderful supplements, you may be tempted to rush right over to your favorite health food store and stock up on all of them. That's not the best idea. Why do I say this? If you have CFIDS, you must remember that part of your problem is malabsorption and maldigestion. In other words, more supplements does not necessarily mean better.

So how should you assess what vitamins with which to start?

* In the first five weeks of treatment, all supplements you take should be aimed at eliminating underlying conditions such as yeast infection, parasites and viruses (see Chapters 5-8). Most of these products, in general, are best absorbed in sublingual (to be taken underneath the tongue) form, followed by powder form, capsules and tablets, in descending order.

During your first five weeks, another goal is the elimination of toxins. So any supplement which aids good bowel movements should be taken. Increase your intake of vitamin C to at least 10 grams a day. Take buffered C to protect your stomach from irritation and add an herbal laxative to your regimen (See Chapter Twelve).

If you take colonic hydrotherapy, now is the best time for those treatments. With your improved diet and killing of micro-organisms, your die-off symptoms (see Chapter Twelve) are at their maximum. Your body needs help to eliminate all these toxins.

One of the most important supplements to add to your program is acidophilus, since it has a great capability to relieve your gastrointestinal symptoms (such as gas, bloating, constipation). Do not add anything else to your supplement regimen during this cleansing phase. Your doctor can assist you in this phase with intravenous administration of vitamin C, intramuscular injections of Kutapressin, AMP and B12, to help you overcome the stressful moments of toxin elimination and the increased fatigue you're likely to experience in initial phases of your treatment.

* Change after five weeks:

After five weeks, your body will absorb nutrients much better. Your improved diet has improved your digestion. So this is the time to add supplement to boost your immune system. Which ones are best?

Antioxidants are a must for everyone, CFIDS and healthy patients alike. Choose either germanium or CoQ 10. If you have food and environmental sensitivities, add vitamin E (800 U.I.) and selenium (100 mcg.) If you have skin problems (dry skin, acne), add beta-carotene (50,000 U.I.) and evening primrose oil (3 capsules of 500 mg. each). Your doctor will be able to assist you in determining what supplements need to be continued to kill yeast, parasites and viruses and to help you in general to achieve better elimination. Make sure you keep on taking acidophilus.

* Remember this Golden Rule:

Don't overdo your supplements. Make sure you know why you are taking each one. If you still have problems digesting and eliminating after the first five weeks, hold off on taking the immune boosters.

Exercise a Must

Have you often embarked on a regular exercise program, only to be discouraged? The U.S. Public Health Service has estimated that only one out of five Americans exercises regularly. It's not that we don't try to exercise. We do. We just give up too soon, because there is too much sweat and hard work to it. We have forgotten how to have fun. And yet, the fact is that there are millions of people dying prematurely because they are totally inactive, and can't maintain a routine as simple as walking three times a week.

The good news is that you don't have to get up at the crack of dawn to huff and puff through your neighborhood. A brisk three-mile walk three times a week is all it takes.

The problem is that most people look at others in considering what is right for them. The stereotype of physical fitness presented to the American public is that of gorgeous young "hardbodies" devoting hours every day to achieving the perfect body. You look at them and ask yourself "How can I ever work out that hard, or look that fit?" After a month of effort, when your body has not metamorphosed into this olympian image, you're resigned to viewing fitness as an unreachable goal. I'll bet that half America's households have stationary bikes and rowing machines, that were bought with great expectations, and discarded after 14 days.

So what is the answer? You must find an exercise that you can ENJOY, and that suits your lifestyle and time schedule. The key to any fitness program is how much you like to actually do it, whether the exercise involved be walking, dancing, playing tennis or jogging. If you enjoy it, you will be so much more likely to stick with it. You are a unique individual and should create a plan that is tailored to your own requirements. Perseverance is the name of the game and maintaining it may be helped by the following proven tips:

• Join a class, or work out with friends. This helps to avoid boredom and will give you an incentive to hang in there because you also feel responsible to your exercise mates

• If you jog, alternate the routes to keep it interesting

• To avoid injury, warm up and cool down by stretching before and after workouts; discomfort and pain are easy excuses for thinking that "exercise is not for you"

• Choose a convenient workout; it often pays to join a health club near your work instead of being stuck in the homecoming traffic; this will allow you to cruise home after exercising, in a much better mood and also in lighter traffic

• Be realistic. Match your program to your fitness level. If you start too low, you may get bored immediately. If you start too fast, you are likely to injure yourself and be discouraged one week into your program. Remember, you're not training for the Olympic Games, so take it easy

• Buy the right equipment, especially when it comes to shoes. Your tennis shoes won't be sufficient to carry you through your aerobic classes. What you need are light shoes designed for aerobic exercise.

Once you understand these simple principles of exercise, it is now time to choose an activity that fits your lifestyle. The smart thing to remember is that you are not in shape when you are only doing one form of exercise. Individual exercises matter less than the ways in which they fit with others. It is wise to choose your own mix and start getting all the parts of your body in shape.

• **Walking** is certainly one of the most appealing activities and it is available to almost everyone. In a high-speed world, a brisk walk offers the gift of slowness. It offers you a true workout, yet allows you time to admire the neighborhood and hear the song of happy birds. You can do it anytime of the day. You don't need a partner (although it does not hurt to have one), and you don't need special, expensive equipment. There are no different levels of competence and it has all the benefits of jogging, without putting so

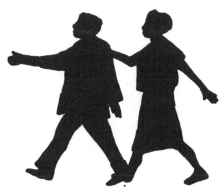

much stress on the joints (there is no better exercise than walking to benefit arthritic conditions). It is the best aerobic exercise, improving your circulation and muscle tone in the legs, while contributing to lower blood pressure and anxiety levels. For CFIDS patients, it is one of the best exercises, since other more rigorous ones may be beyond their limits.

What is a good level, when getting started? How can you gauge the proper exertion level? You should be able to still carry on a conversation while walking briskly, without huffing an puffing. Take a brisk, two-mile walk, and schedule the walks in your calendar (up to three a week) and keep the appointments. Put some vigor into your arm swing, lean slightly forward from the ankles and try different strides.

• **Aerobic dancing** is another popular and pleasurable exercise activity. Aerobic dance classes provide cardiovascular fitness, muscle toning and flexibility. Your lungs increase their breathing capacity and your body becomes more efficient at dissipating heat. Aerobic dancing is a low-impact, long-duration exercise, enough to draw energy from your fat deposits when the dancing last for at least 20 minutes. Aerobic dancing will improve muscle firmness and overall flexibility but will not add great amounts of strength. For those, you may need to add swimming, running or biking to your exercise program.

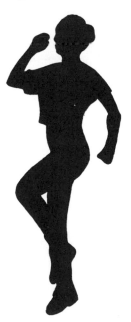

But aerobic dancing is not the only form of dance exercise available. For many Americans, ballroom dancing has become more than an evening out. It is their exercise— recreation of choice. While ballroom dancing is more gentle and low-impact than aerobics, it improves posture, coordination, flexibility, balance and discipline. Dancing with your

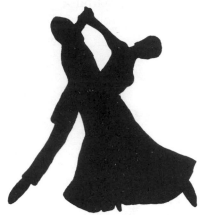

partner requires a level of concentration that will benefit any other sport you do. There is almost no risk of injury and it is not necessary to be in tip-top shape to begin. Dance classes offer a social atmosphere, in a sharp contrast to the "loneliness of the long-distance runner." I know of no better stress reliever and more aesthetically appealing workout than mastering the simple basics of ballroom dancing. Nor is it the sole province of Fred Astaire types. More and more, it is recognized as a workout that puts you in touch with your body, provides a sense of accomplishment, and moreover, will win you admiration from your friends.

• **Cycling** is also high on the list of fitness aspirants. Whether a stationary or a touring bike is used, cycling provides all the benefits of cardiovascular activity, while strengthening the muscles and tendons of the legs. The work provides you with shapely legs without subjecting ankles, knees, legs or backs to jarring impact. There is probably no better exercise to help you recuperate from any knee injury, either before or after an operation. A man riding for half an hour at a 15 MPH, burns 400 calories, not bad when you realize this pace is only slightly higher than a leisurely one. Bicycling taxes the back; the most useful response is to strengthen the abdominal muscles to keep the spine in place.

The three above programs are probably the best for anybody to start with before moving on to more strenuous workouts such as swimming, tennis or weight lifting. The smartest move would be to add to any of the above exercises, a daily stretch or yoga routine. Most of us stretch before workouts, but much more important is stretching after your workout. Anyone can find 20 minutes a day

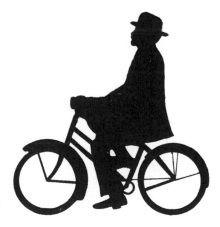

to improve their health and prolong their lives. Within a month or two, you're sculpting a body that is balanced, flexible and strong.

Combatting Indoor Pollution

Living in the Los Angeles area, I am painfully reminded every day of outdoor pollution. On hazy, smoggy days, when the beautiful mountains surrounding our valley disappear from sight, labored breathing, watery eyes, headaches and coughs become a constant reminder of the danger in our air. To avoid these toxic substances in the air, some people go to the beach, the mountains or the desert, but the vast majority prefer to stay inside, in air-conditioned rooms. But is this such a wise alternative? Not if we can believe a report issued in 1984 by the Consumer Product Safety Commission. It states that indoor pollution may be ten times **worse** than outdoor pollution.

Sick Buildings

Let's start with office buildings, where most of us spend the majority of our working hours. Within 30 years, most new jobs will be white-collar positions, with an emphasis on information processing. This means that exposure to indoor pollution will continue. If you're a professional working in an office building, you need to be aware of the following possible hazards in your workplace.

* Inhalants

Poorly ventilated office buildings are at the top of the list. This is a direct result of the energy crisis in the mid-1970s, leading to a trend of energy-efficient design. Newly constructed, airtight buildings reduce heating and cooling costs. However, these buildings rely on recycled oxygen which is not adequately filtered or mixed with fresh air. Because windows are scarce or do not open, workers breathe recycled air full of potentially toxic vapors and cigarette smoke.

What do you inhale?

• Asbestos from insulation, floor and ceiling tiles, especially if the building was erected before 1970. These small dusty fibers can lodge in the lungs, at first irritating and inflaming the lung mucosae, but later, with chronic exposure, resulting in serious and even fatal lung conditions.

• Other pollutants are formaldehyde from glues and fabric, bacterial and viral microorganisms that grow in pipes and ventilation equipment, tobacco smoke and volatile compounds from cleaning and copying fluids and felt pens. The intense light of copying machines turns oxygen into ozone.

• VDT Hazards

Computers, as revolutionary as they have been, have also created new challenges to our health. Video display terminals (VDTs) are everywhere, and yet little is known about their long-range effects on our health. However, short-term consequences are already visible: headaches, skin rashes, muscular pains and depression have been reported by personnel who habitually work in front of VDTs. This is not surprising when we know that these VDTs create an environment of positive ions, which may rob their operators of energy.

• Lighting an Additional Danger

The damaging effects of poor lighting were extensively exposed by John Ott, author of "Health and Light." In spite of dramatic documentation regarding improvement in worker performance and reduction in absenteeism when full-spectrum lighting is installed, very few offices have full spectrum lighting, which contains all the same wave lengths as sunlight. It does not involve much expense to install these lights, but the gain to one's health is enormous. It is important for office workers to lobby for improved environmental conditions.

* What You Can Do

In the meantime, there are things you can do right away to reduce your risk of exposure to dangerous substances. The following is a short list:

• Try to establish a cooperative relationship with your boss, since you're more likely to make changes with his or her blessing.

• Open windows whenever this is possible.

. Bring green plants into your workplace, since they give off oxygen (especially spider plants and philodendron).

• Try to have a shield installed for your VDT.

• Install full-spectrum lights. The cost is only about $ 19. For more information, obtain a copy of "Health and Light," by John Ott (published by Pocket Books, a division of Simon and Schuster).

Toxic Homes

While we have no problems fighting against hazardous waste sites, few of us realize that the risk of getting cancer from exposure to chemicals in water and other solvents found in the home is far greater than the risk from exposure to those chemicals in waste sites. Here is a partial list of the enemies.

* Formaldehyde
* Radon
* Asbestos
* Combustion Gases and Allergens
* Water pollutants

* Formaldehyde

The first product on the list is present everywhere. It is used in the resins to make plywood and wood paneling; in the foam in urea formaldehyde insulation; in the adhesives used with carpeting and wallpaper; in paper products, permanent-press fabrics and hundreds of cosmetics.

Reactions to formaldehyde exposure are well-known: headaches, nausea, dizziness, insomnia, and skin rashes. If you want to measure the formaldehyde level in your home, the 3-M Corporation in White Bear Lake, Minnesota (612-426-0691) sells a device (for around $50) that can measure the amount of formaldehyde in your rooms.

In case the level exceeds the limit that the Federal Government has established, you can apply some simple strategies to reduce the amount of formaldehyde. You can apply an epoxy sealer to plywood and fiberboards already in your house (epoxy is a non-toxic sealer). Another effective move is to buy more house plants, especially spider plants and philodendrons, since they absorb formaldehyde.

* Radon

Decay products of radon are one of the major causes of lung cancer. An odorless and colorless gas, radon diffuses out of rocks and soil and becomes a problem when it accumulates in an enclosed area such as a basement. Radon enters houses through cracks in foundations and basement floors. Again you can test your house for Radon contamination. You can get a measuring device from the "Radon Project, Department of Physics and Astronomy, University of Pittsburgh, PA., 15260. Sealing cracks will reduce the radon levels to some extent, but sometimes a special ventilation system has to be installed.

* Asbestos

This "wonder product" used in almost all buildings between 1920 and 1970 is also highly carcinogenic if fibers are released into the air. Lung cancer and an irreversible lung disease, asbestosis, are consequences. One finds asbestos used in insulation of walls, to strengthen vinyl floors and to fireproof walls. The Federal Government has prohibited its use since the '70s, but many older houses have these sources of asbestos which need to be removed by professionals.

* Combustion Gases and Allergens

The best thing you can do is to get rid of your gas stove and replace it with an electric one. Build up of CO2 (Carbon Dioxide) causes headaches, dizziness, nausea and impaired memory. If you have a gas stove, try to replace it with one that has no pilot light or one that functions through spark ignition. The flames should burn blue instead of orange. If you notice orange flames, then more CO2 gas is escaping into the air. Call your gas company, which will send a repair person to adjust the flame for free. And never try to heat your house with the gas oven door open. Many families have literally asphyxiated themselves in this way.

Another major source of asphyxiation is inhalation of dust particles. Dust contains viruses, bacteria and mites, ready to attack any weakness in your immune system. You have several solutions:

• Negative ionizers and electrostatic precipators are helpful, but no air purifier is as important as keeping your house clean.

• If you have allergies, stay away from dogs and cats, or at least keep them out of the bedroom.

• Wash your bedding, pillows and drapes with 1% tannic acid solution. They will remain hypoallergenic even after repeated washings with detergents.

* Water Pollutants

The purchase of a water purifier will be an investment in your future health. According to the EPA, two percent of the country's community water supply poses a significant risk to human health. If you have questions about the safety of your water, call the EPA's toll-free number (800) 426-4791. One of the problems is to choose the right water purifier for your house. The National Sanitation Foundation, 3475 Plymouth Road, Ann Arbor, MI., 48106, has a list of the most effective ones.

It is clear from the above that we have a hard and sometimes expensive battle in front of us. As more and more people with immuno-suppressed diseases become reactive and sensitive to the environment, the need for "non-toxic" houses will increase. Some architects and contractors are already specializing in this: they use low-toxic or non-toxic materials in particle board, wallpaper glue and paint, and insulation made of cork. The price is about twenty percent higher than for conventional houses, but for the millions of people already suffering from allergies, it is worth it. Considering the cancers and other irreversible conditions toxic house materials cause, it seems a small investment in your health!

Maintaining and enhancing your immunity, if you're already healthy, are always worthwhile goals. Making yourself aware of possible environmental hazards, and taking action, can make the difference in the long run between sickness and health.

REFERENCES
1: Trowell, H. "Fiber: a Natural Hypocholesterolemic Agent." *American Journal of Clinical Nutrition*, 1972: volume 25, pages 464-2: Anderson, J.W. 2: "Medical Benefits of High-Fiber Intakes." *The Fiber Factor*, August 1983. Quaker Oats Company, Chicago.

CHAPTER FOURTEEN

OPEN LETTER TO FAMILIES OF IMMUNO-SUPPRESSED PATIENTS: NINE DAILY CHECKPOINTS TO HELP YOU COPE

"If life seems like one long obstacle course, let poor health not be the chief obstacle."

This chapter contains a message directed to the families of immuno-suppressed patients. And by family, I also mean the extended family: spouses, friends and partners, and even the occasional person these patients might meet at parties or dining occasions. While this chapter mainly addresses the extended family, I hope it also provides a tool for patients. CFIDS patients have to defend themselves continuously against disbelief, rejection and insults about their condition. Laziness, self-centeredness and immaturity are charges leveled at them on every occasion.

The previous chapters have shown to what degree these victims suffer. The family also suffers - they may be frightened, unable to answer the cry for help, or feel manipulated or unloved by the patient.

While knowledge of the disease is a big step forward in securing the support of friends, it takes a lot more to really help: it takes unconditional love. And this was the lesson I learned.

My Own Experience with CFIDS

In my practice I was giving support and treatment to thousands of immuno-suppressed patients. I thought I was doing a good job. I thought I, more than anybody else, understood these patients. I felt empathy for them, I could cry with them, I could feel the desperation they felt. Or so I thought.

I failed to see one thing: I went home after work into an entirely different atmosphere and I lived a completely different life. I could go to the theater, play tennis, go dancing, have dinner with friends... it was all possible. It took my personal involvement in their lives to come to a full understanding of the suffering of both the patients and their families. It was not until I met a friend, S., that I fully understood the suffering of the patient as well as that of the family. Here I was, confronted for the first time, with the reality of CFIDS and environmental hypersensitivity. I realized that the name of the problem was **ENERGY**.

Energy is the one word that dominates the lives of immuno-suppressed patients. They have no energy, and, what's worse, they never know *when* they will have energy. The reasons are various: patients may react to a previous treatment; a woman might be premenstrual; there is suddenly a reaction to a new food; or a man becomes ill from automobile exhaust while driving. In fact, the causes are unlimited, and sometimes hard to pin down. So instead of a whole day, the patient can count on only one-third of the day, the other two thirds being needed for rest, to sit still, waiting for the small rally in mental and physical strength. Sometimes the latter does not come for a whole week, and the daily chores pile up, increasing the anxiety in the patient, especially when the spouse comes home and says: "You had the whole day, what did you do?"

This is the difficult part for the family to understand: the patient did not have the whole day; she might have had two hours of that day. It is very hard for a healthy person to understand this, and it is easy to become irritated with the patient's seemingly "lazy" behavior. But there is no way such patients can push themselves beyond a certain point: they will pay for it tenfold the next day.

So if a patient has two good hours of energy in a day, he or she may feel obliged to use them for everybody and everything else — the long-waiting chores, the friend that absolutely had to see her, the spouse that wanted to see that movie. This leaves no time for their own needs. There are two things dominating their lives: reacting to the disease or the treatments, and spending their remaining energy on everything else but themselves. Not a very easy way to live and not a lifestyle that is conducive to healing. The patient feels worthless and the family feels left out of her world. The disease rules the family.

What Was My Reaction?

I am ashamed to say that I did not do much better than the average person would have done. I could not understand why my friend did not want to be with me as much as I wanted to be with her. Did she not love me as much as I loved her? Sometimes I persuaded her to let me visit in spite of her not feeling well. I finally wore her down by saying, "I'll be there just for you, you don't have to be `up' for me." However, when I was with her, I encountered for the first time the total lack of affection that these patients, who are in crisis, display. She had such a hard time dealing with herself, that there was no room for me or anything else.

I had difficulty understanding that her rejection of me was not personal. I did not understand that her need to rely on me was stressful in itself. Family members take note: those patients do not like the position of dependency that they are put in, they hate it! And although you might think, "I am doing all I can, and I don't deserve this treatment," the patients are the ones who suffer the most. They gladly would trade places with you.

How Did I Get the Help I Needed?

The first help I received was from myself. I wanted to be with S., and I wanted to help her. However, reading some pertinent books she gave me, I began to understand that my "love" was very limited. Sure, I loved her as long as she behaved the way I wanted her to. The moment I had some expectations and she did not read my mind or could not "perform," I was disappointed. My own ego and pain were in the way. In fact, it was my ego that dictated my defensive behavior. Whatever subject came up, I would read between the lines, feel attacked and unloved, and feel justified in retaliating.

I should have known better: the words "attack" and "battle" and even more "ego," leave no place for love. I sensed I was only at the beginning of a road I had never traveled before: the road to unconditional love and inner peace. I knew it was going to be a hard journey, a long process. It taught me several valuable lessons that all of us can use to help an immuno-suppressed patient. I do not presume to force them upon any of my readers; I simply state that I tried to focus on them repeating them to myself every day. I called them my nine daily check points.

The Nine Daily Checkpoints

1. *Practice Unconditional Love*

This is really the primary rule, and certainly the most difficult one to follow. Ninety-five percent of all adult relationships are based on conditions. "I love you, but...," or, "I love you as long as you behave the way I want you to behave." Unconditional love, found in any loving relationship, is the purest form of love. It's more common for parents to love their children unconditionally. It's more of a challenge to love your partner or friend, with all the weaknesses and handicaps that they have, and to accept them for what they are. Of course, this does not mean you should take emotional or physical abuse, which are signs of a disturbed personality.

2. *Love and Forgive Yourself*

If you want to give to the patient in your family, you need to start by loving yourself. You might feel guilty for not being able to help your spouse and find yourself trying to escape the situation. If you are going to forgive and love yourself, you must say goodbye to guilt. You cannot possibly give love if you feel that you do not deserve love.

3. *Forget the Negative Checklist*

I have caught myself many times concentrating on some small negative characteristics of my friend. As a result, small remarks can snowball way out of proportion, causing much more damage than intended. It is so easy to focus on those negative facts, because they allow us to avoid the work needed to improve the relationship. The checklist of faults inevitably becomes bigger and bigger until it takes on monstrous proportions, overshadowing any potential joy. It is helpful during this time to focus instead on the positive points of your partner. Sometimes even in their extreme illness, people can contribute to family society if they are supported in doing so.

Patients should concentrate on their "can do" lists. If they can only perform two tasks a day, they should focus on those instead of drowning in an ocean of uncompleted tasks on the "can't do" list. In this way, patients and their partners and families can save themselves a lot of depression and despair.

4. Have Some Fun With Friends

Family members do occasionally catch the immuno-suppressed disease from the patient. I don't mean physically, but emotionally. Most of the time there is no energy to go to restaurants, enjoy sports or go to parties. Environmental sensitivities exclude an evening at the theater, because your hypersensitive spouse might have a seat next to somebody wearing a heavy perfume. You may start to feel like a prisoner to the immuno-suppressed disease, even though you are perfectly well.

If the patient is able to let his or her partner enjoy time with friends, this can relieve some of the pressure. When two people have room to breathe in a relationship, they are freer to express their love for each other. They don't feel resentful, or blame the partner for keeping them from enjoying life. Having his or her batteries recharged, a spouse can dedicate fresh energy to the patient and actually have more empathy and compassion.

5. Get a Therapist on Your Team

For everyone involved in the family of a hypersensitive patient, a counselor is not only welcome help but a must. The patient needs the chance to unload the frustration of not being able to contribute more to society or family; the guilt he or she probably feels for being such a "pest," and for the mood swings that sometimes elevate to suicidal proportions.

Likewise, the other members of the family need to unload their frustrations, of having to care for a sick person who doesn't seem to be getting better fast enough. The therapist, knowing both parties, can give suggestions. Being non-judgmental and not siding with either one of the parties, he or she will be an intermediary to help establish cohesiveness, which is necessary for the healing of each individual involved.

6. Be Honest With Yourself

The first thing I had to do to cope with this problem was take an honest look at myself. Why did I react the way I did? I caught myself reacting in an insensitive way, as though I did not understand the situation and could not summon any empathy. I could not be the support my friend needed until I first resolved my own issues. This is why a therapist is absolutely necessary; don't think you are smart enough to resolve your own painful issues. It is not a sign of weakness to get some help with your own psychological problems. Understanding yourself will lead to better acceptance of your partner, bring you closer, and strengthen you in handling any future problem.

7. *Give the Sick Person Space*

As already mentioned, energy is the name of the game. If the patients need to withdraw and be by themselves, let them. Don't push them, because then they will have to spend precious energy trying to explain why they cannot accommodate you. No matter what, the result for you will be the same: they will not be able to go along with your desires. For the patients the outcome will not be the same: exhausted because of the efforts to explain, they will require extra time to recuperate — precious time they could have spent with you or on some worthy goal. This necessity for space will vary from person to person, but also from time to time within the same person. During the premenstrual period for women, for instance, the need for withdrawal will be greater.

8. *Be a Team Player*

This is another major rule. You can show understanding by sharing a special diet with the patient. You might be surprised how tasteful it is, how much more energy it will give you, and how pleasant it can be to be innovate. Sharing in this way removes the burden of making two separate dinners. Besides, when patients have cravings, it is no fun for them to see their partners gobbling down forbidden goodies.

Being a team player has some very interesting results. Usually my patients are well-motivated to follow the diet, but some of them receive "static" from their partners for doing so. What happens is that the other person feels guilty about his own lousy diet; it makes him think about it. So if you are someone's partner don't sabotage the diet by buying the wrong foods. Instead, start looking at the healthful food around you and try to develop a taste for that.

Being a team player is not restricted to food intake. Exercise together, stop smoking and drinking, and stay away from drugs. Help the patient organize and execute some of those daily routines; it feels very good to the patient when the daily check-list gets shorter instead of longer.

Even more important in helping the recovery of your spouse is getting tested yourself for candida or Herpes simplex viruses. Patients can work very hard to overcome these chronic conditions, and they relapse because they get reinfected by their spouses. I have seen it happen many times. You can imagine the frustration of patients who feel they are being sabotaged in their hard, long road to personal healing. So be the team player you promised to be when you entered your relationship.

9. Try to Communicate Better

Sometimes patients already feel so guilty that they do not want to express certain wishes. The other partner, feeling repeatedly "rejected," stops asking and assumes that the partner will guess his or her desires. After misunderstanding, anger is the next step. In fact, what happens often is that verbal communication becomes very difficult, because the other party always thinks that there is an "attack," so self-defense is in order.

Adversarial exchanges can lead only to the destruction of any good feeling in the relationship. So if you have come to the point where verbal communication becomes impossible, write each other a letter. And write the whole truth, everything that you would like to express: your anger, frustration, fear, but also your wishes, desires, hopes and love. In fact, make sure you start with the negative feelings, and finish with the positive ones. Be sure the harsh feelings don't outweigh the positive ones.

I hope this "Open Letter" can bring some understanding to all parties. Let's face it. If your relationship survives an immuno-suppressed disease, it will survive almost anything!

What was the outcome of my relationship? I was not able to hold on. In fact, I believe that it is extremely hard to build up a relationship in such situations. How can you get to know each other when you can't do things together? Relationships are built upon common interests, shared pleasures and experiences. It is different when you have already a relationship through marriage before the disease hits. You have known your partner before, there is already a bond. Sadly, a lot of marriages get stranded on the cliff of these diseases. Therefore, this open letter is especially aimed at people in an existing relationship. If immuno-suppressed patients are not currently in relationships, I advise them not to enter one. Both parties will be spared a lot of sadness. Let those patients focus on their recovery — they will need all the energy they have left.

CONCLUSION

Some people may still believe that immuno-suppressed conditions are diseases of the future. It must be clear by now to the readers of this book that they are already reality for millions of people.

But there is one positive aspect of this situation: it may force a change of attitude in the medical profession. Suddenly there is no "magic bullet" available to wipe out these strange diseases. The variety of symptoms puzzles the medical community. "It is a fad disease." "A good psychiatrist is what you need." — these are some of the initial reactions mainstream physicians have had to the baffling complex of symptoms experienced by these patients.

Such patients will no longer tolerate such insults, but instead will seek the help of true healers, finding the support they need and deserve.

It is also clear that the task of facing these immuno-suppressed diseases is a formidable challenge for the patients. I think that their biggest mistake is that they make the disease the "absolute ruler" in their lives, to whom everything else must give way. Acting this way causes the patient to lose control over their lives, so that they cannot commit themselves to the true goal of recovery.

Often the lack of self-esteem sets up a dangerous pattern of guilt. First, patients feel guilty because they cannot participate in a constructive way in family life. More money is spent on special diets, doctors' visits and medications, funds that could have been used for more "meaningful" purposes. On the other hand, non-compliance with the diet, and cutting out exercise evoke more guilty feelings for patients, putting them in a double-bind, no-win situation. Patients need to set realistic, positive goals, accepting the challenges facing them.

Another obstacle between the patient and his recovery is the way we habitually view medicine and its therapeutic modalities. We are used to getting immediate responses to a treatment: we take a pain pill, and the discomfort disappears rapidly. We can't sleep, but we are given a sleeping pill that allows us to get the necessary rest.

We are accustomed to knowing the approximate length of time before our disease runs its course. Healing a fracture will heal in four to six weeks; flu symptoms will last about a week, and so on. This is perhaps the most frustrating aspect of the immuno-suppressed diseases. "How long is this going to last?" and "When will I be feeling better or cured?" are the most frequently asked questions.

These questions have no quick and easy answers. Too much depends on the willingness of the patient to change his or her life style. Most of the time the patient is battling several immuno-suppressed conditions at the same time. Moreover, patients generally tend to underestimate these conditions. That makes them impatient and irritable, emotions not very conducive to boosting the immune system! We have to learn to look at each step of improvement, and not try to jump to the end point, a goal we cannot see.

You cannot ask your doctor to predict the future. Your doctor is human and a valuable partner in your efforts to fight your disease. Instead of looking forward, look backwards at the course of your disease. Hopefully, you will begin to see that you are already accomplishing more than you did one week, one month, or even one year ago. Seeing your progress in this perspective can stimulate you to continue on instead of stalling in self-pity and despair.

As outlined in previous chapters, immuno-suppressed diseases have no single known cause, so that the dream of a single cure for them is just that, a dream. Western medicine has an obsession with "objectivity." We have become increasingly technical, forgetting that medicine remains an art, where the true healer has to master his technique in the same way as a great artist does. We must not forget that there is an important interaction between healer and patient. It will become even more evident in the future that emotions are one of the most important factors in triggering diseases that affect our lives.

Illness in one part of the body does affect the whole. If doctors fail to treat this unity, they will be treating the patient improperly and incompletely. You cannot subdivide human beings into small parcels and believe that all those magnificent technical advances will structure a perfect creature.

True healing is giving, without restraints of peer pressure and personal desire such as making quick money. The true healer in the future will fuse in his practice ancient methods (acupuncture, homeopathy) with new technical advantages, but always with one goal in mind: he will give himself to the patient with his whole heart and with compassion.

I would like to close this book with Hippocrates' "Advice for the Physician."

"Sometimes give your services for nothing, calling to mind a previous benefaction or present satisfaction. And if there is an opportunity of serving one who is a stranger in financial straits, give full assistance to all such. For where there is love of man, there is also love of the art. For some patient, though conscious that their condition is perilous, recover their health simply through their contentment with the goodness of the physician. And it is well to superintend the sick to make them well, to care for the healthy to keep them well, also to care for one's self, so as to observe what is seemly."

I hope that from this book you've gained a new understanding of health and wellness and that with the tools provided here, you have what you need to truly achieve peak immunity and be full of life.

APPENDICES

APPENDIX 1: CFIDS SYMPTOMS

If patients have several of these symptoms present in each category, especially when doctors have difficulties making a diagnosis for these "unexplained" symptoms, then the doctor should think about CFIDS as a possible diagnosis. This list should be used in conjunction with the self-scoring questionnaire in Chapter One.

A. Brain Symptoms
Difficulty in concentrating —— Anxiety attacks
Decreased short-term memory —— Suicidal thoughts
Drowsiness —— Frequent Headaches —— Severe mood swings
Depression —— Excessive Anger and Irritability —— Frustration

B. Hormonal symptoms
PMS —- Difficulties getting pregnant —— Early Menopause
Flare-up of yeast infection week before menstrual cycle or immediately after intercourse —— Loss of Sexual Desire or Impotence —— Endometriosis —— Menstrual irregularities (No menstrual cycle, prolonged or shortened menstrual cycle)
Vaginal discharge —— Vaginal burning and/or itching

C. Digestive symptoms
Gas —— Abdominal distension —— Frequent Diarrhea
Constipation —— Hemorrhoids —— Mucus in the stools
Greenish stools —— Anal itching —— Inability to lose weight

Bad breath —— Constant hungry feeling —— Food allergies
Presence of white-yellow fur on tongue —— Cravings for sugar, bread, and carbohydrates

D. Other symptoms
Recurrent colds [More than 5-6 in one year] —— Cannot hold chiropractic adjustments —— Constant Fatigue —— Recurrent sore throats and swollen glands —— Cold limbs
Itching [Anal, vaginal, or all over the body] —— Joint and muscle pains
Insomnia [Most of the time for at least several weeks] —— Hives —— Intermittent low-grade [99.5F] fever
Dizzy spells —— Earaches and recurrent ear infections
Chronic sinusitis —— Blurred vision —— "Floaters"** in eyes—-
Nocturnal sweats —— Recurrent bladder infections —— Severe itching——Numbness, tingling and feeling of pins and needles in limbs—— Nosebleeds —— Hematomas

** The presence of "floaters" in the vision IS a sign that warrants checking out by an ophthalmologist, but if no reason is found, it can be part of CFIDS, relating to toxin build-up in the liver.

If you have 3-4 symptoms in each of the above catagories, you would do well to consult with a doctor.

APPENDIX 2

AUTOBIOGRAPHY OF A YEAST CELL

For a long time, most illnesses were linked to viruses, bacteria or parasites. Rarely were fungi suspected. However, radical changes in our diets, environment and lifestyles have made immuno-suppressed conditions a number one condition on anyone's list. Once the immune system is suppressed, the greatest opportunist in our body, candida albicans, senses that decreased strength immediately and starts multiplying with devastating effect. This chapter is intended to present the life history of a candida albicans cell, to lighten your heart by helping you give your enemy a face. In that way, you may be more equipped to vanquish that enemy. As the late Norman Cousins believed, laughter is an essential ally in the battle against disease.

Hi! My name is candida albicans, but anyone hardly calls me that. You know how it is. Mom and Dad get carried away when they're choosing a name, then find out that nobody's going to call you by your full name anyway. So you can call me "yeast" — all my friends do. If you want to address me in more formal company, the name "fungus" will not offend me. I am going to tell you my life story just to set the record straight. You see, lately, I have gotten a bad rap because of those New Age "holistic doctors," as they call themselves. So many books have been written about me, depicting me as an evil monster, that I am glad to finally have the chance to tell my side. After listening to my case, I hope you will recognize me for what I am: a happy-go-lucky friendly character, meaning no one pain or harm.

Let me begin by telling you that I have been around as long as you have—that is, since human beings began inhabiting this earth. Of course, I was not always as popular as I am today. Before the modern era, I stayed mostly in the background, and frankly that's what I prefer. I don't need all the hoopla. All I really want to do is get along and live with you in peace. Thanks to all the sweets and antibiotics, I underwent a personality change, and now, like Dr. Jeckyl and Mr. Hyde, I have a split personality. When I'm fed sugar I get greedier, and I want to conquer the entire human world.

I must say, I have a devilishly humorous streak in me. Every month, with a lot of women, I have a five day carnival time, called the premenstrual period. During that time, I issue a loud demand for huge chocolate bars. And boy, it is like the song of the Sirens: women feed me all the chocolate I can handle. You can imagine what that does to them when they eat all that candy. They cry, they are hurt, they are angry, they become irritable and impossible to live with. But look at the bright side. It gives men a valid, legitimate reason to leave home for a while, and women a deserved break.

Over the years I have made many, many friends. One extended family is Virus, ubiquitous foe of human beings. Undoubtedly, Virus is my strongest cousin. Medicine still has not figured out how to attack him, and luckily, not enough attention has been paid to Vitamin C, one of his enemies. The greatest breakthrough of my career came with the discovery of the "miracle drug" Penicillin in 1940, the first member of the Antibiotic family. Thanks to modern scientific medicine the Antibiotic family grew rapidly. Every year, several new family members joined the dynasty: Tetracycline, Sulfamide, and Vancomycin.

Few people appreciate what Antibiotics have done for me. They attacked those frontier guards of the colonic plantation, Lactobacilli, bifido bacteria and Bulgaricus. These meddling busy bodies kept on saying to me, "Don't grow so fast, there is a place for everyone here in the colon." Now, that was holding a wet blanket on one guy's fast growing ambitions—namely mine, and it didn't please me one bit. So I made a deal with the Viruses: "Attack humans, have a ball and display all your little tricks." It worked wonderfully. Viruses invaded, causing sore throats, little coughs, running noses—and people demanded the Antibiotic dynasty to come to the rescue. Of course, the Antibiotics—while attacking bacteria—had great respect for my partner Viruses and in no way harmed them. On the other hand, it wiped out those spoil-sport bacteria and allowed me to grow.

I must admit, I have learned some tricks from my other friends too, even Bacteria, who told me once: "Produce green mucus, and Antibiotic will be summoned, no questions asked!" I still thank Bacteria for that hint. Or, "Go and hide in the sinuses, and cause some congestion." It is amazing how this works, everytime. You know how beneficial this is for Bacteria? Antibiotic loses its potency by trying to attack Viruses and when finally, the Bacteria do show up, they are resistent to Antibiotic and can freely roam throughout the body. One favor begets another!

I must tell you, too, that we yeast cells are a very close knit family. Even when we die, we find ways to support each other. Our dead bodies are called "Toxins." Our funerals are beautiful and lengthy. We try to stay as long as possible in the human body after our own deaths (we recognize a good thing when we have it!) and find it exciting to be able to choose from so many exits on our way out to life after death. Can you imagine: we can choose between nose, mouth, eyes, skin, anus and vagina. But our favorite is the bladder. Our corpses are able to produce a burning, irritating sensation in the bladder. Guess who gets the blame? Bacteria. They don't mind, that's what good friends are for.

Of course, as soon as Bacteria are expected as the culprits, that other old friend Antibiotic appears on the scene, and we are in business again. Life (and even death) can be sweet. And please, don't try colonic hydrotherapy or enemas: I am sure you would not like to be washed out rudely and be carried off in a hurry when you just passed away. What's the expression: "Rest in Peace?" "Let sleeping dogs lie?"

I would be dishonoring my closest relative, Parasite, if I did not mention him. You think I am a big eater? Think again. Parasite has that wonderful trick of increasing people's appetites. That gimmick is almost as good as my premenstrual carnival time. Parasite has also made many friends. Many people in undeveloped countries have accepted Parasite as a host in their bodies, no questions asked. Of course Parasite is grateful. To show his gratitude, he doesn't cause discomfort in his friends, the "chronic, asymptomatic carriers." He stays inside them peacefully until he is ready for his "out of the body experience." Parasite loves to travel. Being the Californian of the microcosmic world, he moves easily from one human house to the other, causing "Montezuma's revenge." Frankly, we could care less what it is called—the name sounds good and there is always an ample supply of unsuspecting bodies available.

Of course, with my popularity, you can imagine that I have created a few enemies. Among these, is the "holistic doctor" I already mentioned. They call themselves "Yeastbusters," and if you ask me, they are living in Fantasyland. They say that I am

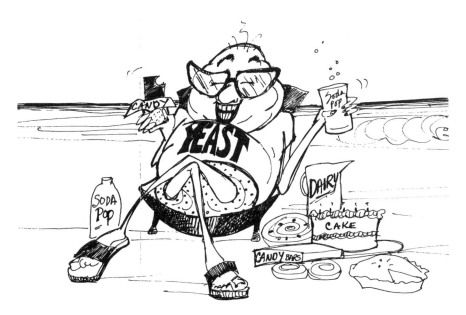

The yeast cell living the high life, when fed by a diet rich in processed sugars. The first step in eliminating overgrowth of yeast is to "starve the candida" (see Chapter 9.)

responsible for more diseases than you can shake a stick at, and they threaten to expose all my little tricks. I don't appreciate that. Especially when most doctors ignore me altogether. As I said, I'm shy and prefer secrecy. But the Yeastbusters think that they can control me by helping my other foes, the White Blood cells, with vitamin supplements which they give to their patients. Who needs vitamins, after what I've taught you? Didn't I not teach you how to add preservatives, hormones and antibiotics to your food? You know my favorite slogan, "All types and colors welcome." So, Yeastbusters get off my back, will you!

There is no way that you'd find me in Mrs. Gooch's or those other healthfood stores. Hey, who wants those foods with silly names, such as Amaranth and Quinoa when there is delicious hamburger, beer, wine and peanuts. You can see that nobody deserves to wave the American flag more than I do, since those are my all-time favorite foods. I am the all-American boy.

You know what my favorite saying is? "An apple a day keeps the doctor away." You see, an apple is considered healthy by the yeast loving doctors, but it ferments and makes me grow faster than ever. This is truly a conspiracy between the doctors and me.

As much as anyone else in this world, I deserve my vacations. Of course, some people think I have too many of those days, but let's face it, I am a hard working fellow. My most exciting period of the year is between Halloween and New Year's. Between these two wonderful events there is Thanksgiving and Christmas. Those four holidays are engraved in gold in my memory. There is so much love and cooperation between Human Beings and us that it brings tears to my eyes. No matter what diet people are on, during that time my allies and I get the most wonderful foods, the ones that make us burst with energy—us not you! Sugar, cakes, alcohol, champagne, wine, chocolate—too much to mention, my mouth is watering at the thought. Oh! I almost forgot Easter. You know, people always expect the Easter Bunny to bring them baskets full of chocolate and candy, I mean the real good stuff. Well, very few among you know that the name Easter Bunny originally started as "Yeaster" Bunny, but according to our policy of avoiding overexposure, and to help people in general to overcome their guilt feelings about porking out over these goodies that we yeast cells, disguised as bunnies, bring around, our P.R. person thought it was a good idea to accept the name Easter Bunny. That brings me to my favorite way of traveling: a cruise! Can you imagine, they feed you every 22 minutes, you can't turn your head without food being thrown at you. You know all these cruise lines deserve to be brought under one banner: SS YEAST LINE.

And just like any of you, we yeast cells are partial to certain Human Beings. The type we love the most—in fact we created, is the Worrier, the Type A Personality. You know the one that is a compulsive obsessive, analytical, the anal-fixated type who wants everything to be sparkling clean. Worry or stress depresses our enemy, the Immune System, and gives us an opportunity to grow. These chronic worriers are truly our friends. So a song like, "Don't Worry, Be Happy" is on the bottom of our hit parade. I tell people to view this song for what it is: an anti-candida aria, disgusting and truly revolting. I hate that song. These are the songs that are on our Top Ten: "Sugar Baby," "Sugar Shack," "The Candy Man," "Lollipop," and "Smoke Gets in Your Eyes." Sweet, aren't they!

Like many other health-oriented people, I have a standard set of diet rules, known as the "Yeast Lifetime Diet." I expect the book to become the number one best seller as soon as it hits the stands. I know these rules will be very beneficial for you and I want you to post them on your refrigerator door. So here they are:

* Ban all bathroom scales and never consult a doctor who has one in his examining room.

* Eat all you want of everything you like. Keep the refrigerator door and your mouth open most of the time.
* Eat all you want—swallow and don't chew.
* The best thing to eat—more.
* Every time you get the urge to exercise, lie down until it passes.
* The maximum exercise allowed is browsing leisurely through shopping malls.

Any other suggestion for exercise should be met by the phrase: "I don't have the time." An alternative is skipping through your TV programs using your remote control, while absorbing our latest invention, the TV snacks. Refuse to buy TV's without these remote devices. Ride your bike from your dining room to your bedroom. And stay in the bedroom as long as possible.

I knew you would appreciate these golden yeast rules. I hope I have encouraged you to start a fan club. Make sure only to admit people to the club who love chocolate, fats, ice cream and those who hate fitness programs.

O.K. So you are going to see some pretty disgusting guidelines in this book. I advise you not to follow them because they teach you to give up goodies such as sugar and chocolate. You don't want me to stop wreaking havoc on your system, do you? There is so much more still to tell you, but I have to run. I just got invited to a birthday party, and there is still time to contact all my hungry cronies. You know what I'm going to find there? Cake, chocolate, champagne and beer. Way to go!

I hope that the above story will brighten your spirit as well sharpen your vigilance against the overgrowth of the yeast cell.

To anyone suffering from yeast overgrowth, I strongly advise to consult my previous book on the subject, "**Candida, the Symptoms, the Causes, the Cure,**" available in health food stores and which can be ordered by writing to the following address:

Luc DeSchepper, M.D.
2901 Wilshire Boulevard, Suite 435
Santa Monica, California 90403
(213) 828-4480

APPENDIX 3

HELP IN COPING WITH BUREAUCRACY

Must Financial Hardship Be a Companion of Chronic Disease?

You Can Get Help

For anyone with a chronic illness, the need to work creates a double-bind. First, the fear of being out on the streets forces people to keep their jobs rather than seeking the help and time off to restore their health. The emotional and physical stress endured by the patients often is enough to push them over the edge, prompting a sudden absence from work. By that time, however, patients will be in much worse shape than if they could have taken off when they first needed to.

Secondly, once patients have made the decision to stay at home, to fully concentrate on their recovery, they find out that bureaucracy in our free world is no easy horse to tame. They are in for a shock when they try to apply for disability. I have seen this in my practice so many times, because CFIDS patients have run into this problem more than anyone else. To these patients, who are chronically tired, have difficulties concentrating, thinking and reasoning, the process of filing for disability looks like an endurance test.

Above all, CFIDS patients have been denied their disability because the Social Security Administration makes decisions based on "medically accepted" diagnoses. Up until 1991, that meant tough luck for these patients. Their doctors were called "quacks" and patients were diagnosed by the Social Security doctors as suffering from "somatization of psychological problems," or in other words, "depression."

So what can you, as a patient, do? Prepare yourself as if going to a war. Just as we are not sending our soldiers without weapons and preparation to the battlefield, you should arm yourself with some expert advice. Be aware of one thing: the Social Security system makes their regulations so strict, that only the people who persevere, will get what they deserve in the first place. In these days of recession and budget deficits, bureaucrats are often instructed to be even more stringent. Unfortunately, patients do give up, and often on their first application, which is what Social Security counts on. But a high percentage of patients win their disability cases at later administrative stages, so it's important to persist in the fight for your rights.

You better get some help on your side: an experienced attorney and your doctor. Not just any attorney will do. You need one experienced with disability law because the Social Security decisions are based on a complex set of laws. Just telling the Social Security Administration that you are too sick to work will not always do.

However, your doctor will be crucial when it comes to being successful in your application. And it does not hurt if you can help him or her along with suggestions on how to write the right letter. It helps to understand that disability is defined as "experiencing a physical or mental impairment or combination of such impairments which have lasted or can be expected to last for at least twelve months; the impairments must be totally disabling." As we know, the successful performance of a job requires the ability to *sustain* the physical requirements of work (lifting, sitting, bending, standing...) as well as to *sustain* the mental requirements of work (attentiveness, concentration, short-term memory). Anyone suffering from CFIDS recognizes his or her limitations in the above rule. For you and your physician's benefit, I have compiled a "model letter" that can be used in the application for Social Security benefits.

Model Letter to Apply for Social Security Benefits

To: Social Security Administration
     Bureau of Disability Determination

TO WHOM IT MAY CONCERN,

Ms. or Mr. Jane/Jim DOE has been a patient in my office since.... S/He was diagnosed as suffering from Chronic Fatigue and Immune Dysfunction Syndrome (CFIDS).

This syndrome shows symptoms and signs that are equivalent to those set forth in the Organic Mental Disorders.[OF DSM-III?], all of which Ms. DOE still suffers at this point:

* Signs of Organic Mental Disorder (12.02):

1/ Memory impairment: short-term with inability to learn new information 2/ Disturbances in mood with severe mood swings 3/ Emotional lability with attacks of sudden crying 4/ Marked difficulties in maintaining social functioning 5/ Difficulties in concentration resulting in frequent failure to perform tasks in a timely matter.

Looking at the above restrictions, Ms. DOE is unable to sustain any competitive employment. The above symptoms strike at random and without warning, making it impossible for any of these victims to plan or to get involved in any work relationship, even on a part-time basis.

* Signs of Affective Disorder (12.04):

1/Depressive syndrome with insomnia, irritability, difficulties in concentration, decreased energy (constant fatigue) and feelings of guilt and worthlessness 2/ This situation results in marked restriction of activities in her/his daily living, deficiencies in concentration resulting in failure to complete tasks in a timely matter, and marked difficulties in maintaining social functioning.

A successful performance of a job in this field of work requires not only the ability to sustain the mental requirements (which as outlined above patient does not fulfill) but also requires the ability to sustain the physical requirements of work. Ms. DOE is not able to perform basic work activities such as standing, walking, lifting, bending, sitting, talking, hearing, and use of judgment on a continuous basis.

Ms. DOE has experienced the above symptoms to an extreme degree. Having always been an outgoing person, very socially oriented, and ready to perform any demanding task, these aspects of her CFIDS syndrome are especially hard for her to bear. It is extremely important for any professional judging a CFIDS patient on her physical and mental capacities to perform, to understand the fluctuating, irrational course of this disease. Affected people can feel and look wonderful at 10 a.m. and look and feel horrible at 2 p.m.

It is my conclusion that Ms. DOE is totally disabled and unable to perform even sedentary work. Detailed medical and immunological evaluations and physical examinations constitute the basis of my professional conclusion. Following the diagnostic guidelines for chronic fatigue syndrome established by Holmes, et al., in the March, 1988 Annals of Internal Medicine, Ms. DOE has undergone sophisticated tests to rule out any other possible disease at this moment.

There is no doubt about this patient's diagnosis. However, there are no clinical means available to adequately measure the extent of disability and individual variability in this regard. Ms. DOE has unsuccessfully attempted low stress exercise and activities many times, but, as for most people with this syndrome, any activity results in a worsening of her symptoms. Restricting activity is, at present, the only way to prevent exacerbation of these symptoms. Ms. DOE is not able to undertake any work at this time beyond her own self care. The delicate balance sustaining her fragile plateau can be easily upset by stress of any kind—emotional upset, job frustration, work demands or overexertion. The additional stress will create an intensification of any of these symptoms. Those of us who have been treating patients with this illness for some time now recognize that although the complete etiology of the disease remains unexplained, we are dealing with something very serious and potentially devastating.

Ms. DOE's laboratory results are enclosed. She is receiving (name medications). Her last visit was on ..... Her prognosis is guarded and a date to return to work cannot be predicted. If I can be of any further help in supporting Ms. DOE's disability, please let me know.

Sincerely yours,

Dr. X

A letter such as the above is helpful not only for obtaining Social Security benefits, but can also bring considerable clout when your case has to come to court and you have to convince the administrative law judge of your entitlement to benefits.

INDEX

A

B

B-cells, 31, 36-37, 48-49, 61, 64
Barnes basal temperature, 46
Beta-carotene, 185-186, 191
biofeedback, 181
birth control pills, 9, 43, 71, 80, 186
Blastocystis hominis, 83, 88, 95
brain fog, 25, 65, 74-75, 142, 144
breast implants, 28
bruising, 46
Bueno-Parish test, 86
burning vagina, 56, 173

C

candida antibody test, 47, 55, 71, 78
capryllin, 131
carbohydrate cravings, 156
carnitine, 158
CFIDS symptoms, 24, 39, 44, 134, 170, 210
CFIDS triggering factors, 21-22, 28, 136
chromium, 159
climate, 11, 24
CMV, 47, 62-63, 66, 69-70, 108-109, 125
coenzyme Q10, 188
colon cancer, 2, 24, 183
colonic irrigation, 175
cortisone, 9, 26, 37, 52, 80, 137-138, 172, 189
cryptosporidium, 83, 88
cycling, 194
cystitis, 51-52, 56, 74, 77, 81, 172

D

dampness, 106
depression, 11, 22, 24, 51-54, 65-66, 73, 75, 84, 91, 109, 125,
    143-144, 148, 153, 156, 158, 169, 171, 181, 196, 203, 210,
    218
diagnostic tests, 39, 44, 72, 136, 177
die-off symptoms, 132, 144, 173, 190

Giardia lamblia, 82, 86-89, 91, 95
grapefruit seed extract, 93

H

Hahneman, 138
headaches, 12, 25, 54, 64, 75, 91, 141-142, 171, 174, 195-198, 210
health food stores, 131, 182, 217
Helper T-cells, 31, 36, 47-49
hereditary factors, 19, 79
herpes simplex, 26, 39, 47, 49, 61, 63-64, 69, 91, 94, 96, 107-109, 125-126, 134, 143, 206
Herxheimer reaction, 64
homeopathy, 137-140, 146, 209
hydrotherapy, 174-175, 190, 214
hypoglycemia, 5, 19, 51, 53, 72
hypothyroid, 46
hypothyroidism, 81

I

immune panel, 47, 49
interleukin-2, 49, 112, 115
interstitial cystitis, 51-52, 56
ITL, 55, 68, 70, 87

K

Kutapressin, 126, 190

L

lactose-intolerant, 133
laxatives, 174
lecithin, 144-145
Lifestyle, 2, 17-18, 26, 39, 60, 102, 113, 119, 137, 142, 152, 178, 191-192, 201
Lyme disease, 49, 51, 54-55

M

magnesium, 53, 126
mercury dental fillings, 26
mitral valve prolapse, 57
mononucleosis, 60, 62-63
multiple sclerosis, 6, 45, 51, 62, 95, 107, 172, 219, 221
MVP, 57-59

N

neurotransmitters, 145, 160
Nizarol, 130-132, 141
Nutrasweet ™, 2, 8, 22, 164
nutritional factors, 8, 22, 79
Nystatin, 130, 134, 141

O

oat bran, 149
oils, 149-150, 160-162, 166
olive oil, 162, 166
organic, 25, 150-151, 166, 188, 220
Overeaters Anonymous, 147

P

parasites, 29, 45, 47, 53, 66, 81-89, 93-95, 108, 123, 136-137,
        163, 165, 169, 190-191, 212
Pau D'Arco, 56-57, 129, 142, 167, 173-174
penicillin, 26, 56, 80, 213
pesticides, 10, 23, 25, 150
phagocytes, 30-31, 36, 138
pinworms, 84-85, 89
pollution, 25, 195
polyzym, 189
premenstrual syndrome, 13, 158, 210
Prozac, 136, 143-144
purged stool test, 47, 78, 85-86, 92

R

radon, 197
retrovirus, 63, 69-70, 105
rheumatoid arthritis, 5, 19, 21, 37, 189
roundworms, 84, 87

S

saccharin, 2, 22
serotonin, 24, 143, 160
shigellosis, 89
sick buildings, 195
Sinequan, 125, 136
SLE, 49, 52
Social Security, 218-219, 221
spastic colon, 73
spirulina, 186
stool cultures, 84, 86, 93
suppressor T-cells, 36, 47-48, 125
sweeteners, 22-23
synthroid, 46
systemic lupus erythematosus, 37, 51-52

T

Tagamet, 125
tapeworms, 85, 88
taste, 2, 22-23, 74, 86, 134, 148, 158-159, 205
thymus, 19, 31, 187, 189
toxin buildup, 169-171, 173, 211
toxin elimination, 190
toxin exits, 172-173
triggering factors, 3, 5, 15, 17, 19, 21-22, 28, 63, 69, 72, 74-75, 78, 127, 137, 145, 177
Type A personality, 216
tyrosine, 144, 160